A HANDBOOK FOR

TRAINEE NURSING ASSOCIATES

A HANDBOOK FOR

TRAINEE NURSING ASSOCIATES

EDITED BY

Neil Davison and David Matthews

Lantern

ISBN: 9781914962042

Lantern Publishing Ltd, The Old Hayloft, Vantage Business Park, Bloxham Rd, Banbury, OX16 9UX, UK
www.lanternpublishing.com

www.cla.co.uk

British Library Cataloguing in Publication Data
A catalogue record for this book is available from the British Library

The authors and publisher have made every attempt to ensure the content of this book is up to date and accurate. However, healthcare knowledge and information is changing all the time so the reader is advised to double-check any information in this text on drug usage, treatment procedures, the use of equipment, etc. to confirm that it complies with the latest safety recommendations, standards of practice and legislation, as well as local Trust policies and procedures. Students are advised to check with their tutor and/or practice supervisor before carrying out any of the procedures in this textbook.

Cover design by AM Graphic Design Ltd

Typeset by PageMajik Pvt Ltd, India

Printed in the UK by Ashford Colour Press Ltd

Last digit is the print number: 10 9 8 7 6 5 4 3 2

CONTENTS

PREFACE

Registered nursing associates are important members of the modern healthcare team. The *Handbook for Trainee Nursing Associates* provides relevant theory to support trainees on their level 5 educational programme and towards registration with the Nursing and Midwifery Council (NMC). It will also be the foundation for their future practice as nursing associates. Each chapter is linked to the outcomes of the NMC's *Standards of Proficiency for Registered Nursing Associates* (2018) and uses activities and examples to apply theory to contemporary practice.

Neil Davison
David Matthews

Acknowledgements

Our thanks must go to Lynne Bedson, a colleague and lecturer with considerable experience of teaching healthcare students. Lynne raised the idea of a book like this and its value to trainee nursing associates over coffee and informal chats.

ABOUT THE AUTHORS

Linda Bale

Linda is a Senior Lecturer and Course Lead for the Nursing Associate programme at the University of Worcester. As a Registered General Nurse, she has experience over a diverse range of clinical settings, including working as a research Sister for Cancer Research UK. She has a Master's in Education (MEd), a Postgraduate Certificate in Teaching and Learning (PGCert) and is a Fellow of the Higher Education Academy (HEA). Linda is committed to widening participation in Higher Education and supporting nursing students to reach their full potential.

Neil Davison

Neil worked in trauma and orthopaedics after the completion of his state registration and orthopaedic nursing qualifications in the 1970s and early 1980s. He lectured at Bangor University for two decades where he was made a Teaching Fellow in 1999. He has presented papers nationally, published in journals and has written a book on clinical calculations and numeracy, now in its second edition.

Josh Hodgson

Josh is a Senior Lecturer in Learning Disabilities at Teesside University. A second-generation nurse, he's been working in the field for around 15 years and has been a Registered Nurse in Learning Disabilities (RNLD) for just over 10 years. Josh has worked predominantly in the private sector across a range of services including learning disabilities, mental health, end of life care, clinical assessment and management. He is currently studying towards his doctorate and is examining perceptions of the field of learning disability nursing with a view to uncovering people's experiences and increasing understanding.

Graham Jones

Graham is Senior Lecturer in Nursing at Teesside University School of Health & Life Science. He is also a board member of the UK charity Transform Healthcare Cambodia, which supports the development and enhancement of healthcare provision in Cambodia. Graham is in the final year of study for a Professional Doctorate.

Anneyce Knight

The late Anneyce Knight, who died in 2021, had retired earlier that year from her role as Associate Dean for Global Engagement and Senior Lecturer in Adult Nursing at Bournemouth University, where she was also the Programme Leader for the Return to Nursing Practice course. She qualified as a registered nurse in 1982 and worked in orthopaedics and oncology, then trained as a midwife. She continued to practise in a variety of nursing and midwifery clinical settings before moving into Higher Education in 2000. Prior to taking up her role at Bournemouth University in 2015, Anneyce was the Course Lead for the innovative Foundation Degree in Health and Social Care (clinical) for Associate Practitioners, a joint NHS and Southampton Solent University collaboration. Previously she was at the University of Greenwich, where she held a number of positions. She was passionate about the need for compassionate care, thereby enhancing the quality of patient care, particularly at the end of life. Her primary research interests focused on public health and wellbeing, areas in which she published and presented nationally and internationally.

David Matthews

David is a Lecturer in health and social care at Bangor University, and is programme leader for its BA Health and Social Care, where he teaches issues and subjects relating to the social determinants of health and health policy, as well as supervising undergraduate and postgraduate dissertations. His research interests and publications focus on critical and materialist understandings of the welfare state and social policy, with a particular emphasis on the impact of neoliberalism and capitalism for physical and mental health. In addition, he has an interest in the development and evolution of Welsh health policy during the era of devolution.

Nevin Mehmet

Nevin is a Senior Lecturer and Deputy Head of the School of Human Sciences in the Faculty of Education, Health and Human Sciences at the University of Greenwich, London. She has an MA in Medical Ethics and Law and currently teaches ethics across a range of programmes, including public health, paramedical science, social work and health and social care. Her main research interest lies in the areas of values and ethical decision-making within paramedic practice.

INTRODUCTION: BACKGROUND AND CONTEXT

Two decades of change

Since the turn of the millennium the National Health Service (NHS) has been subject to significant organisational and structural changes. Among the many changes, arguably some of the most significant which have impacted upon the establishment of the Nursing Associate (NA) role include the consequences of devolution to Scotland, Wales and Northern Ireland, resulting in differing health policies implemented throughout the United Kingdom. Additionally, the growing expectation that greater numbers of healthcare professionals should be educated to degree level has radically altered the professional status of many. Where once there existed a great division between those who were required to have a degree qualification and others where practical skills were thought more relevant, such as existed between doctors and nurses, now it is increasingly recognised that for effective care to be provided at all levels, academic knowledge and practical skills are equally important. Furthermore, *Agenda for Change*, implemented in 2004, constituted a significant reconstruction of occupational roles within the NHS. This divided the workforce into nine bands based upon equivalent skill sets, qualifications, responsibilities and pay scales (Matthews, 2015). Of particular significance, it introduced Band 4 level professional roles.

RECAP

Over the last two decades the NHS in Britain has experienced significant organisational change. There are many reasons for this, but three of the most important include:

1. Devolution to Scotland, Wales and Northern Ireland, meaning that different healthcare policies throughout the UK result in different ways the NHS is organised
2. More healthcare professionals expected to be educated to degree level
3. Introduction of Band 4 professionals.

Professional boundary evolution

All professions experience change over time, with the roles and expectations of people occupying professional positions changing to meet differing circumstances and pressures. The healthcare profession is no exception. Evolving boundaries between healthcare professionals and changing expectations of individuals who occupy them has been a feature of healthcare for more than a century (Nancarrow and Borthwick, 2005). Being a nurse today, for example, is very different to what it was a hundred years ago. This is as a result of the significantly different ways healthcare is organised in the UK, as well as very different external pressures placed upon the delivery of healthcare, such as various social and economic forces. During the last two decades changing expectations of how healthcare professionals perform their roles has dominated debate within the NHS and influenced greatly how care is delivered, with this having been experienced no more so than by nurses.

RECAP

Expectations as to what roles and tasks professionals in the NHS perform and carry out in their roles, have changed during the last twenty years. Registered nurses have experienced significant change. Over the last two decades the reasons that nurses have experienced great changes in role expectations have been influenced by varying pressures, but include:

1. Declining numbers resulting in a skills shortage (Wakefield *et al.*, 2010; Spilsbury, Adamson and Atkin, 2011)
2. Reductions to junior doctors' hours
3. Growth of older population and increased demand on the NHS
4. Government economic policies (Matthews, 2015).

As a result of these developments the practice of many has expanded to that of advanced practice levels (RCN, 2012), contributing to the growth of nurse practitioners and clinical nurse specialists (Kessler *et al.*, 2010). Subsequently, nurses have increased their involvement in (Spilsbury and Meyer, 2005):

1. Prescribing rights
2. Triage in A&E
3. Pre-operative assessments.

The result of these developments has been an advancement of their skill base (McGuire *et al.*, 2007). Their role has become characterised by more complex medical tasks (Wakefield *et al.*, 2010). With the transformation of the nursing role, the status of healthcare assistants (HCAs), situated at Bands 2–4 of the NHS career framework, has been enhanced, primarily as a result of having absorbed various practices associated with nursing (Cavendish, 2013; Kessler *et al.*, 2010; Matthews, 2015).

RECAP

Professional expectations of registered nurses have grown during the last two decades, and they perform more complex medical tasks than they previously did. As a result, there has been an increased emphasis upon healthcare assistants situated at Bands 2–4 performing tasks which were once the domain of nurses.

Growth of healthcare support roles

Increasingly throughout the NHS, HCAs have experienced an expansion of their responsibilities and duties due to tasks being delegated to them. Many HCAs sit at Bands 2 and 3; however, during the 2000s attention was focused upon enhancing support roles situated at Band 4, one band below registered nurses. Initially this emerged with the development of the Assistant/Associate Practitioner (AP). Established in 2002, the AP role was gradually introduced throughout the UK, but largely in locations where funding allowed, rather than where a need was identified (Henshall *et al.*, 2018).

Considered as higher level support workers, the main objective of the AP was to support registered professionals (Henshall *et al.*, 2018) by being equipped with skills and knowledge usually thought greater than that possessed by traditional HCAs situated at Bands 2 and 3. In order to obtain this level of knowledge and skill base, as well as reflecting wider expectations that greater numbers of health professionals should be educated to degree level, AP education was based upon practitioners obtaining a foundation degree qualification (Matthews, Davison and Bedson, 2014; Matthews, 2015).

RECAP

Initial efforts to provide support to nurses occurred with the development of the Assistant/Associate Practitioner situated at Band 4. Not restricted to clinical settings, AP positions developed in such diverse settings as (Henshall *et al.*, 2018; Millar, 2011):

1. Acute and community nursing
2. Occupational therapy
3. Learning disabilities
4. Radiography
5. Adult mental health
6. Health visiting
7. Paediatrics.

Occupying an intermediate position between HCAs at Bands 2 and 3 and Band 5 professionals, difficulties emerged, however, with regard to clarifying the role (Mackinnon and Kearney, 2009). In part this was as a result of the role not being registered or regulated.

With a lack of clarity as to how to define the AP, varying definitions emerged. On the one hand Spilsbury *et al.* (2008) considered the AP as being a higher level support worker, while Wakefield *et al.* (2010) argued they should be thought of as advanced nursing assistants. Nonetheless a lack of clarity regarding the boundaries between APs and Band 5 professionals defined the role (Allen, McAleavy and Wright, 2012; Henshall *et al.*, 2018; Millar, 2011; Whittingham, 2012), with APs potentially engaged in different duties depending upon where they practised in the UK.

> ### RECAP
>
>
> The AP role was never regulated, nor was it a registered position. The result was a lack of clarity as to its purpose. With the AP being found in many clinical and non-clinical settings, what holders of the role did was not standardised and would vary around the country.

The nursing associate

The AP continues to be a part of the NHS, but arguably it has not become as embedded as was envisioned. Nonetheless, the need for a professional role, one which in particular assists registered nurses, remains as relevant as ever if the NHS is to continue to provide effective patient care. It is within this context that the nursing associate (NA) was introduced. Launched in 2016 in England (at the time of writing it has not yet been introduced within Scotland, Wales and Northern Ireland), situated at Band 4, the stated objective of the NA is to bridge the gap between existing HCAs and registered nurses (Glasper, 2017).

> ### RECAP
>
>
> Nursing associates were introduced in 2016 to fill the gap between HCAs and nurses. Crucially, the NA is not considered an HCA, but as an extra source of providing nursing care. This was made very clear by the Nursing and Midwifery Council (NMC) who argued:
>
> "The role will contribute to the core work of nursing, freeing up registered nurses to focus on more complex clinical care."

As a professional source of support for nurses, the NA is only to be found within acute and clinical contexts. However, there is no restriction on which settings they will practise in, being located within the four domains of nursing:

1. Adult nursing
2. Mental health
3. Learning disabilities
4. Children's nursing.

RECAP

A nursing associate is not a higher-level HCA, but an extra tier of nursing professional. To be equipped with the skills and knowledge to provide effective care, in a further recognition of the value of higher education to be an effective practitioner, all NAs must be educated to foundation degree level. The academic value of the NA qualification is greater than many of the registered nurse programmes which existed prior to 2010 (Glasper, 2017), after which time qualification as a registered nurse required a degree. In an act which illustrates clearly the centrality of the NA role to the provision of quality care and its status within the wider NHS, the NA role, unlike that of the AP, is regulated by the NMC. Not only does this mean that NAs will be held accountable as all professionals should, but this is also important for NAs to obtain national professional recognition, as well as ensuring the public have confidence in them.

RECAP

In order to support nurses, all nursing associates must obtain a foundation degree designed to train students to become a nursing associate. Once qualified, they will become registered health workers within the NHS.

References

Allen, K., McAleavy, J.M. and Wright, S. (2012) An evaluation of the role of the Assistant Practitioner in critical care. *Nursing in Critical Care*, **18**(1): 14–22.

Cavendish, C. (2013) *The Cavendish review: an independent review into healthcare assistants and support workers in the NHS and social care settings.* Available at: https://assets. publishing.service.gov.uk/government/ uploads/system/uploads/attachment_data/ file/236212/Cavendish_Review.pdf or bit.ly/3mfrtlc (accessed 22 December 2022).

Glasper, A. (2017) Nurse education and the development of the nursing associate role. *British Journal of Nursing*, **26**(1): 56–57.

Henshall, C., Doherty, A., Green, H., Westcott, L. and Aveyard, H. (2018) The role of the assistant practitioner in the clinical setting: a focus group study. *BMC Health Services Research*, **18**. Available at:

https://bmchealthservres.biomedcentral.com/articles/10.1186/s12913-018-3506-y or bit.ly/3kAOCOq (accessed 22 December 2022).

Kessler I., Heron P., Dopson S. *et al.* (2010) *The Nature and Consequences of Support Workers in a Hospital Setting.* NIHR Service Delivery and Organisation Programme. Available at: https://njl-admin.nihr.ac.uk/document/download/2027291 (accessed 22 December 2022).

Mackinnon, I. and Kearney, J. (2009) *Assistant Practitioners: scoping exercise. A report to Skills for Health.* The Mackinnon Partnership.

Matthews, D. (2015) Assistant practitioners: essential support in a climate of austerity. *British Journal of Nursing,* **24**(4): 214–17.

Matthews, D., Davison, N. and Bedson, L. (2014) Foundation degree, a pathway to practice: mentors are magic. *British Journal of Healthcare Assistants,* **8**(10): 506–510.

McGuire, A., Richardson, A., Coghill, E. *et al.* (2007) Implementation and evaluation of the critical care assistant role. *Nursing in Critical Care,* **12**(5): 242–9.

Millar, L. (2011) *The Role of Assistant Practitioners in the NHS: factors affecting evolution and development of the role.* Skills for Health.

Nancarrow, S.A. and Borthwick, A.M. (2005) Dynamic professional boundaries in the healthcare workforce. *Sociology of Health Illness,* **27**(7): 897–919.

RCN (2012) *Advanced Nurse Practitioners: an RCN guide to advanced nursing practice, advanced nurse practitioners and programme accreditation.* Royal College of Nursing.

Spilsbury, K. and Meyer, J. (2005) Making claims on nursing work: exploring the work of healthcare assistants and the implications for registered nurses' roles. *Journal of Research in Nursing,* **10**(1): 65–83.

Spilsbury, K., Stuttard, L., Adamson J. *et al.* (2008) Mapping the introduction of assistant practitioner roles in acute NHS (hospital) trusts in England. *Journal of Nurse Management,* **17**(5): 615–26.

Spilsbury, K., Adamson, J. and Atkin, K. (2011) Challenges and opportunities associated with the introduction of assistant practitioners supporting the work of registered nurses in NHS acute hospital trusts in England. *Journal of Health Service Research and Policy,* **16**(Suppl 1):50–6.

Wakefield, A., Spilsbury, K., Atkin, K. and McKenna, H. (2010) What work do assistant practitioners do and where do they fit into the nursing workforce? *Nursing Times,* **106**(12): 14–17.

Whittingham, K. (2012) Assistant practitioners: lessons learned from licensed practical nurses. *British Journal of Nursing,* **21**(9): 1160–7.

STUDY SKILLS

Neil Davison

This chapter relates to all of the *Standards of Proficiency for Nursing Associates* (NMC, 2018), as the ability to access, read, interpret and apply knowledge underpins all areas of nursing practice.

LEARNING OUTCOMES

When you have completed this chapter you should be able to:
- Identify the strengths and weaknesses of your study skills.
- Appreciate how you prefer to learn.
- Organise your study time to keep on top of the nursing associate course.
- Confidently find and accurately read information relevant to your course.
- Make accurate and clear notes.
- Make the most of structured learning activities like tutorials, lectures and seminars.
- Prepare to write assignments and take examinations.

1.1 Introduction

Congratulations on achieving a place on a nursing associate education programme! Your study skills are evidently good enough to have got you this far, but you need to be certain that they will support you over the next two demanding years and throughout your career as a nursing associate. There are significant challenges in your course, such as relatively short periods of study, longer periods of clinical placement and shift rotas, that make demands on your ability to engage with academic work. Nursing associates need to know how to learn, as they are required to develop their professional knowledge and skills prior to registration (NMC, 2018). This chapter will help you to develop your study skills to meet the challenges ahead.

1.2 Check your study skills

Modern healthcare courses use a variety of methods of learning. Some methods may be more traditional, such as lectures, tutorials and practical demonstrations, while some take advantage of developments in technology to support simulations, online lessons and discussions. The methods used to assess student progress also vary from essays, reports, dissertations and care studies to examinations. Nursing associates are also assessed on their competence in the clinical environment. This broad spectrum of ways of learning and assessment means that you have to take an honest look at your study skills. Thinking about how you study is the first stage of getting organised to deal with these challenges.

ACTIVITY 1.1

Rate your study skills competence using the headings below:

Study skill	Good	Satisfactory	Could be improved
Self-organisation & time management			
Finding and reading information			
Effective note-taking			
Participating in a: • tutorial • lecture • seminar			
Preparing for: • assignments • examinations			

Using your own results as a guide, you might want to continue to read through this chapter or focus on the areas where you need most development by going directly to the relevant section.

1.3 Learning preferences

ACTIVITY 1.2

Spend a few minutes thinking about the way you like to learn about a subject; maybe consider something that you needed to learn as part of your job or a previous course.

Do you like to read information from a textbook and make notes?

Are you more inclined to recall information if it is on a chart, graph or picture?

Do you prefer to discuss information?

Are you a 'hands-on' learner, remembering best when you have taken part in an activity?

These questions can help indicate your learning style and might help you to study during your nursing associate course.

- If you find seeing information presented on charts, pictures, graphs or PowerPoint slides easier to understand and recall, you may be a 'visual learner'.
- If discussing information, listening to instructions or repeating information to another person are your preferred ways of understanding, then you might be classed as an 'auditory learner'.
- A preference to read information in books or journals and take notes suggests that you might be a 'read/write learner'.
- Preferring to touch and feel objects and having practical involvement indicates you may be a 'kinaesthetic learner'.

How individual students prefer to learn has been debated widely in the literature and is referred to as a learning style. Knowing your learning style can be helpful but it shouldn't restrict you or prevent the use of different strategies. It is worth remembering that a preference for a particular approach to learning does not automatically mean it is the most effective one for you, so keep an open mind.

1.4 Getting organised

When you received the news that you had achieved a place on the nursing associate course, you probably experienced a mixture of emotions; elation, joy, relief. Fairly swiftly your mind may have focused on the practical realities about the course: placements, assignments and exams. You may have had a few moments of self-doubt, asking yourself questions like 'will I be good enough?' and 'will I be able to do the assignments?'.

Don't spend too long thinking about what you may perceive as your weaknesses. Learning to become a nursing associate involves several fundamental components:

- Practical skills
- Underpinning theory
- Professional skills, behaviours, standards and attitudes.

Being accepted onto a nursing associate course means that you have already demonstrated your motivation and ability to achieve these. The selection process considers your qualifications, communication skills and any job or work experience. Many jobs entail learning new skills, and modern employers expect staff to demonstrate the behaviours and attitudes that reflect the values of their organisation. If you have achieved these in a previous job, there is no reason to doubt that you can learn the practical and professional skills expected of a trainee nursing associate. The theoretical knowledge required for registration will be taught to you during your course and applied to your clinical placements. If you have previous healthcare-related experience, you will

>> **As a trainee nursing associate you need to become an independent, self-motivated learner.**

have learnt some without realising it. During initial introductory training for a role in the healthcare setting or clinical observation and physiological measurement courses, you will have been introduced to basic anatomy and physiology. Identifying the normal range for body temperature, blood pressure and heart rate and how these are controlled is some of the knowledge that you will build on during your course.

Studying to become a nursing associate involves a commitment to put time aside to ensure your success. Module lecturers and your personal tutor will advise you what is expected but you are the one who has to organise the time, find resources and information and meet assignment deadlines.

1.4.1 What you can expect from your module lecturer or personal tutor

What they will do:
- Discuss your ideas about an assignment and how you plan to develop it
- Provide feedback on a specified amount of the written assignment; on some courses lecturers will be allowed to read a specific number of words or percentage of the assignment, while others may be able to read a draft copy
- Identify strengths and weaknesses in your work, focusing on key aspects:
  - does the assignment address the title?
  - is it written in a style that is readable and fluent?
  - are the discussions appropriate, developed in a logical manner and do they have support from appropriate evidence?
  - are references and evidence cited correctly?

What they don't do:
- Chase you to make appointments
- Tell you what to write
- Tell you what grade they will give your assignment
- Correct every spelling mistake or grammatical error
- Proofread your assignment
- Demand an assignment from you; this may seem harsh but as a trainee nursing associate you need to become an independent, self-motivated learner for your future career.

What you need to do:
- Arrange appointments with your module lecturer to submit assignment work, and to meet and discuss the feedback; this can be done face to face, by phone or email

- Make sure you submit assignment work by the agreed deadlines
- Keep your assignment within the word limit
- Reference accurately to avoid plagiarism.

Plagiarism is the use of another person's information without acknowledging them as the source. The information could be an essay, textbook, journal article or website. Universities view plagiarism very seriously and use computer software to detect it. This may result in a reduction of the grade awarded to your assignment or the assignment being classed as a fail; you might even be deemed to have failed the course or expelled from your university. Universities have the same view of 'academic essay writing services', more commonly known as 'essay mills'. Irrespective of how professional and supportive they claim to be, they are suppliers of essays, written by someone else for a fee. Remember that you are studying for a qualification that enables you to work in a position of trust, and honesty forms the basis of trust.

Recognising that you haven't got time to do everything that you want to is an important part of organising your studies. If you focus on your studies, it is also the case that what you have to do doesn't all need to be done at the same time. There are three steps to getting organised that will help ensure you make the best use of your time and meet deadlines.
- Prioritise what needs doing
- Set goals to identify what is to be done and by when
- Develop a plan to act as a reminder.

1.4.2 Prioritising

ACTIVITY 1.3A

Make a list of all the study-related activities that you need to achieve.

A typical list in your first year might read like this:
- Read an introductory chapter on nursing & pharmacology before first module lecture later this week
- Book time in skills laboratory to update CPR skills before start of year 2
- Arrange to meet with Health science module lecturer to discuss plan for assignment due in 3 months
- Read 3 articles for Evidence-based Practice assignment, due in 6 weeks
- Make a revision plan for drug calculation exam at start of year 2
- Write reflection on last clinical placement to keep portfolio up to date – should have been done by end of last week
- Arrange to meet with mentor on next clinical placement starting in 4 weeks
- Start to develop plan of Evidence-based Practice assignment, due in 6 weeks

- Find suitable nursing & pharmacology book in library
- Do a literature search for Evidence-based Practice assignment.

ACTIVITY 1.3B

Mark each task in your list as A, B or C:

A = Very important

B = Important

C = Not very important

Go through your B list and decide which of these are really A or C.

Go through your A list numbering each item, starting with 1 as the most urgent, 2 less urgent and so on.

The A list in priority order will look something like this:

1. Write reflection on last clinical placement to keep portfolio up to date – should have been done by end of last week
2. Find suitable nursing and pharmacology book in library
3. Read an introductory chapter on nursing and pharmacology before first module lecture later this week
4. Do a literature search for Evidence-based Practice assignment
5. Read 3 articles for Evidence-based Practice assignment, due in 6 weeks
6. Arrange to meet with mentor on next clinical placement starting in 4 weeks
7. Arrange to meet with Health science module lecturer to discuss plan for assignment due in 3 months
8. Start to develop plan of Evidence-based Practice assignment, due in 6 weeks.

These items have been relegated to the C list:

- Book time in skills laboratory to update CPR skills before start of year 2
- Make a revision plan for drug calculation exam at start of year 2.

1.4.3 Setting goals

Using your prioritised A list, set dates for completing each item. This sets targets to aim for but you do need to be realistic, bearing in mind other demands on your time such as shopping or attending your children's parents evening at school as well as your work-based learning. Goals need to be achievable, so if you can't achieve them, break them down into smaller steps.

1.4.4 Develop a plan

Recording your goals and target dates on a timetable, wall planner or in the calendar on your smartphone will not only act as a reminder but will give a sense of achievement as you make progress through your study plan.

When planning ahead, it is easy to focus on the coming weeks but don't forget to look at the demands on your time for the remainder of the semester and throughout the academic year.

Things to watch out for:
- Assignment submission dates
- Several assignments that need to be submitted close together
- The start of new modules – you may have to do some preparatory reading to gain the most from classroom content.

Remember that time spent sleeping, relaxing, working and exercising is as important as time spent studying. Balancing time for your studies and time for life, family and friends is critical to keeping healthy. When you need encouragement and support during your course, it is usually family and friends who provide this as well as practical help like childcare or cooking meals, so don't neglect them.

The nursing associate course lasts for two years so if possible you need to find a permanent place to study, not the dining room table. Having to set up before you can start studying and tidy up at the end of each session wastes time and becomes a burden. Your study area needs to be away from disturbances and distractions, with connectivity for your computer and a place where you can have your study plan displayed.

Allocate regular time for studying; something like blocks of two hours are ideal with short breaks taken every 20–30 minutes. You will need to allocate one hour to review your notes and carry out additional reading for each hour of classroom time, but you will speed up over time. Don't be tempted to set aside one or two entire days to work solidly on an assignment; this isn't productive and will exhaust you mentally and physically.

1.5 Finding and reading information

1.5.1 Finding the information you need

To develop your understanding and support your assignments and practical work, you will be expected to be able to find the appropriate information, academic or scholarly sources. Once qualified, you will be expected to keep your knowledge up to date. Scholarly sources have usually been reviewed by experts for accuracy.

Scholarly sources could be:
- Books
- Journal articles
- National Institute for Health and Care Excellence (NICE) guidance
- Government policy and reports.

You can search online for additional information – patient organisations like Diabetes UK or the Royal Osteoporosis Society are invaluable sources of information targeted at both patients and professionals.

You will be expected to evaluate all of the information used in your work, especially that obtained from the internet.

When using websites, ask:
- Who owns or runs the website?
- Why was the site created?
- When was it last updated?

If you find a website that appears to offer the model answer to your assignment question, keep well clear as it is likely to be an essay mill which will charge for providing an essay. You are then left to face charges of plagiarism and academic misconduct.

A good starting point is your module reading list. This gives information about key resources like textbooks on the subject that are suitable for your level of study. Reading lists usually include articles published in journals. Books and journals will be available through your university library as hard copies or online as ebooks and ejournals. University library search facilities, searchable databases of up-to-date healthcare-related journals and e-resources are accessible online, saving time and possibly travel. At the start of your nursing associate course it is vital that you work through the library tutorial or attend a workshop to become proficient in finding information. Librarians are specialists in finding information, so don't be afraid to ask for advice. Once you have found journal articles or books related to your module subject, these will also refer to books and journal articles published earlier.

1.5.2 Effective reading

Having identified and located information, reading through it in a timely manner is essential. As well as providing information for your practice and assignments, reading will help to improve your own style of writing. Well written material is easier to read and communicates a clearer message than a wordy and cumbersome style of writing. Students who read widely and effectively frequently achieve higher grades.
- You may have to read an article or chapter several times to gain most benefit from it.
- Initial reading helps you to gain an understanding of a subject.
- Additional reading develops your understanding, offering ways to apply your knowledge and may introduce alternative theories about the subject.

A technique for developing your reading skills is SQ3R: Survey, Question, Read, Recall & Review.

Survey:
- When you first read a piece of text, survey.
- Don't attempt to read every word or make notes.
- Read the introduction or contents page to judge how relevant the text is to your needs.

Question:
- Is it worth reading?
- Which parts are relevant to my area of interest?
- How will this help my studies?

Read:
- Identify sections to carefully re-read and parts to skim read.
- Re-read the relevant parts in more detail:
  - developing an understanding of the key points
  - writing down definitions of unfamiliar terminology.

Recall:
- Make notes.
- Apply the new knowledge to your assignment.

Review:
- Do this an hour or two after the initial read-through.
- Repeat the survey, read and recall stages to make sure you have not missed any key points.

1.5.3 Effective note-taking

Making useful and meaningful notes is one of the foundation stones of both your academic and clinical work. Notes taken in the classroom will be the roots of your understanding of the subject, while those taken from journals or books may act as the basis for an assignment. In the clinical environment, your notes may form part of patient records.

Note-taking is useful:
- As a learning aid to help focus your reading
- To help develop the skill of putting ideas into your own words, demonstrating understanding and interpretation of a subject
- As a method of finding information for an assignment or exam revision.

How to take notes

There is no one method of note-taking that suits all students, and the style that you choose may reflect your preferred learning style. In a lecture you do not have time to write down every word that the lecturer says. When taking notes from a journal or textbook, you may have the time but you need to read and interpret the key points of the text and record it in a way that you understand. When you return to them when writing an assignment or revising for an exam, they must be meaningful, clear, concise and accurate and cover the key points.

One common method of note-taking uses headings, subheadings and bullet points; for example:

The cardiovascular system

Contains: blood vessels & heart

Blood vessels
- Arteries
  - carry blood away from the heart
  - 3 layers
    - endothelial lining
    - middle layer smooth muscle & elastic fibres
    - outer coat
- Arterioles
- Capillaries
- Venules
- Veins

Some students prefer diagrammatic styles that start with the core issue written in a bubble, adding bubbles as the subject expands, branching outwards but making links between related bubbles.

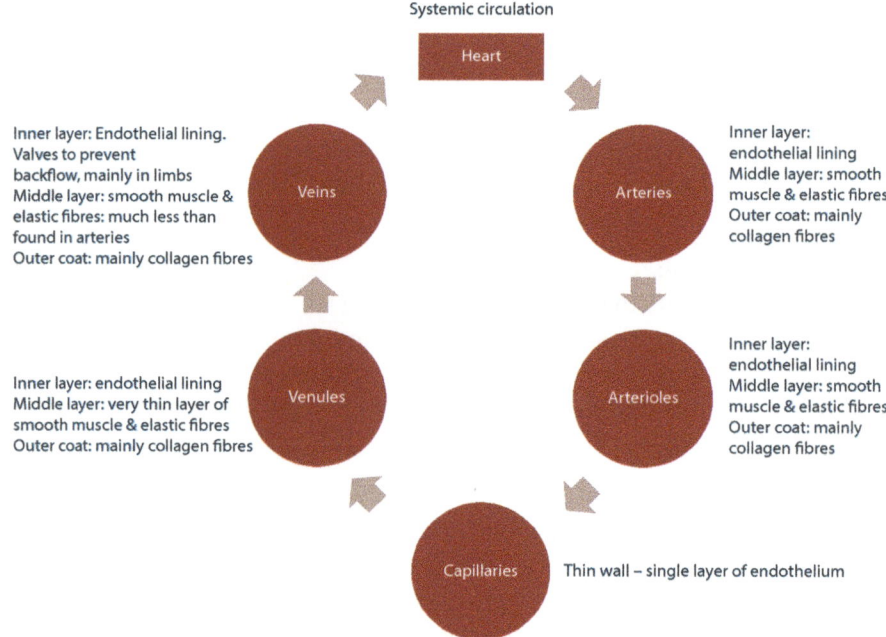

Figure 1.1 *Example of diagrammatic style of note-taking.*

1.6 Participating in specific learning and assessment activities

1.6.1 Tutorials

At the start of your nursing associate course you will be allocated a personal tutor and will be expected to attend tutorials with them. Usually these are gatherings of a small number of students from the same group. Tutorials are part of your professional education like lectures and practical demonstrations, so don't expect to be able to sit quietly in the corner.

Tutorials usually take the form of a discussion based on a contemporary health issue, recent assignment or an agreed topic and aim to:
- Increase your understanding of a subject
- Challenge your ideas and views about a subject.

Preparing for a tutorial

If the tutorial is based on a recent series of lectures or assignment, make sure that you attend these or read through your assignment. If you have been directed to any reading material in preparation, read it through and make notes.

Participating in a tutorial

A tutorial will allow you to:
- Share ideas with other students
- Hear differing views and opinions on the topic
- Increase and clarify your understanding

Challenge or change your ideas
- Develop your critical thinking skills
- Increase your confidence speaking in a group.

Taking part
- Present your views supported with evidence, in a brief and clear manner.
- Listen respectfully to the views of other students even if you strongly disagree.
- Let other students speak and don't interrupt.
- Build on what other students have said.
- Don't be afraid to give honest opinions.

1.6.2 Lectures

Lectures are a traditional method of teaching students in one group. In some subjects, groups can be as large as 500. Lectures have been considered to be a passive form of student learning but technology has given students more interaction, with the use of electronic voting systems allowing the canvassing of student views, opinions and understanding. Frequently, lectures are broken down into smaller blocks of learning, starting with a short lecture-style presentation and including video clips and possibly group work.

Preparing for a lecture

A lecture is likely to introduce you to new information that may be the foundation for future tutorials, seminars or assignments. It is likely to be information-heavy and demanding on your note-taking skills.

Participating in a lecture

A lecture will:
- Allow you to obtain information on a new subject
- Provide an opportunity for you to clarify difficult concepts in the subject.

Taking part:
- Find out which module learning outcomes the lecture will address.
- If you are new to the subject, read an introductory chapter in a recommended textbook and look up any new or unfamiliar words in the glossary or a dictionary.
- Check the title of the module assignment, as the lecture may provide key information for this.
- Check the module on the university virtual learning environment; lecture notes and presentations may be available to read through before the lecture.
- Note any references given during the lecture and follow these up afterwards; make sure you integrate them at the correct point in your notes so they make sense when you use your notes for revision.
- Make notes that you can expand after the lecture.

1.6.3 Seminars

Seminars are an active method of learning, usually in small groups of between 12 and 20 students. No two seminars will be identical but frequently they comprise two parts: the presentation by the seminar leader then an opportunity for discussion and questions.

Preparing for a seminar

In a seminar there is an expectation of some knowledge of the topic, so allow sufficient time to read or complete any learning activity before the seminar.

Seminars focus on a specific topic and aim to allow you to gain a deeper understanding of the topic through active participation.

Participating in a seminar

A seminar will allow you to:
- Explore values and attitudes
- Develop critical thinking skills
- Develop analytical skills
- Increase your confidence in presenting your views.

Taking part:
- Complete any reading or preparatory work or you will not benefit from the seminar.
- Check for any ground rules such as confidentiality.
- Find out if questions are welcome during the presentation or later.
- Listen carefully to key issues presented by the seminar leader and any questions they pose.
- Consider how the ideas presented fit with your understanding based on your reading, preparation and clinical experience.
- Consider the views and opinions of other students based on your preparatory reading around the subject.

1.6.4 Writing an essay-style assignment

There are three issues to consider when writing an essay-style assignment:
- The layout
- The content
- The structure.

The layout

Advice on how your essay is laid out and presented will be provided by your university. There is usually an online guide which will tell you:
- Which typeface, font size and line spacing to use
- What information you must include on the title page
- Where to display your candidate number
- If the essay needs a contents page
- How and when to submit your essay, online or as a paper copy.

The content

Reading the essay title or question is the starting point for writing your assignment, but don't rush into writing yet. Have a copy of the title displayed where you study, to avoid drifting away from the main issues.

You need to:
- Read the question
- Underline the verb that tells you how to answer the question
- Underline the key ideas and issues.

ACTIVITY 1.4

Identify the verb and underline the key issues in the following essay title:

"Discuss the role of critical reflection for nursing associates"

This essay requires an answer presented as a <u>discussion</u> on the key issue of <u>critical reflection</u>.

Similarly, if the title of your essay reads "Discuss the importance of person-centred care", you have to answer the question using a <u>discussion</u> on the key issue of <u>person-centred care</u>.

The following table gives the definitions of verbs commonly used for written assignments as well as exam papers.

Verb	Definition
Assess	Estimate the value of something, considering positive and/or negative aspects
Compare	Look for similarities and differences between two or more issues/concepts
Define	Write down the precise meaning of the word or phrase in detail
Describe	Give a detailed account
Discuss	Examine by argument; sift and debate, giving reasons for and against
Evaluate	Similar to Discuss, but with a judgement in the conclusion
Explain	Give detailed reasons for a principle/attitude/concept
Outline	Indicate the main features of a topic / sequence of events
Summarise	Give a concise account of the main points of the issue. Leave out details and examples

About 60% of the time you spend writing an essay will be used to think, read and plan. All of this needs to be completed before starting to write.

Think about what you already know about the subject of 'person-centred care'. You may have covered this in lectures or have experience of it from clinical practice, so note any key issues that you are familiar with. For example, you may know that it is claimed to improve the quality of care and to help individuals develop a healthier lifestyle. Looking out for these issues in the literature helps to focus your reading.

Reading about 'person-centred care' is the next stage. Returning to the essay title "Discuss the importance of person-centred care", you will need to define 'person-centred care' as well as discussing the importance. Check through the module reading list and your lecture notes for references relating to person-centred care; this is the starting point for your reading. This reading material will also have references to other sources, so find and read these.

To obtain recently published journal articles, you need to perform a literature search through your university library.

Make notes in your own words as you read through the evidence and keep a careful record of the reference details so you can construct an accurate reference list for the assignment. Sometimes questions arise during your reading; for example, 'what evidence is there that person-centred care helps to develop healthier lifestyles?' Note these and follow them up in your reading. Finding and presenting alternative viewpoints is an essential part of a discussion.

Construct a plan that outlines the issues that you plan to address and the order they will appear in your assignment. Indicating which evidence from your reading will be used to support your various discussions will make life more straightforward when writing the assignment, as you'll know which notes to refer to.

A plan might look like:
- Definition:
    - putting people at the centre of services they receive (Jones, 2021)
    - help people to receive care when they need it (Brown, 2019)
    - helps people to take care of themselves more (Brown, 2019)
- Develop healthy lifestyle (Jones, 2021)
- Promotes service user involvement (Makepeace, 2020)
- Improves quality of care (Williams, 2018)
- Reduction in service use (Comrie, 2019)
- Receiver of care is more of a partner in care instead of passive recipient (Graham, 2021).

This is the time to start writing your essay, initially in draft form. Once completed, re-read, edit, refine and proofread your work to convert it into an assignment ready for submission.

RECAP

When writing an essay-style assignment:
- Read the question
- Identify key verbs and issues
- Think
- Read and make notes
- Plan the essay
- Write a draft copy of the essay
- Edit, refine and proofread.

The structure

The introduction to an assignment should tell the reader how you are going to address the question and let them know what the essay will cover.

The main body of the assignment is where the issues are discussed, supported by the evidence from your reading.

The conclusion to the assignment should include all of the main points made within the essay, without repeating them word for word, and needs to answer the essay title. Finally the conclusion should draw together your ideas within several sentences, in a similar manner to a judge summing up the evidence in court at the end of trial.

It is essential that after your hard work you have an assignment to submit. Regularly save your work to a backup hard drive, data stick or online storage like Google Docs. Remember that portable hard drives and data sticks have a limited working life so if in doubt, use a new one. You can always send a copy of your assignment to yourself via email – that way there is always an up-to-date copy of your work stored safely.

Checking your written work

Proofreading and checking your academic work for errors is difficult. You already know what you intended to say and what the sentence means so are unlikely to spot every mistake. It is important that the meaning of your written work is clear so that an examiner can follow and understand your discussions. This skill is transferable to your practical work, as patient records need to clearly communicate the care needed by patients and their response to care received.

>> **Proofreading is a useful skill that will be transferable to your practical work.**

Read your work through carefully and slowly – some students prefer to print an essay when they are proofreading. Don't rely too much on a spell checker as it will not spot words spelt in error, like 'too' and 'to', and 'form' instead of 'from'. Reading your essay backwards will give you a better chance of identifying typos and spelling mistakes as there are no discussions to distract you. Jargon-free short sentences are easier to understand than long, clumsily written ones. Reading textbooks and journal articles will help to develop your style of writing.

Check through your written work and ask yourself:
- Have I put my ideas in the right order or are they random and mixed up?
- Have I supported my ideas with evidence?
- Do I lead the reader through my work with signpost words like 'however' and 'therefore'?

- Do my paragraphs contain one idea and do the sentences in the paragraph support or link to that idea?
- Do I link each paragraph so that the essay flows or do they read as separate blocks of text?
- Does my conclusion include all of the main points that I made within the essay?
- Does my conclusion answer the essay title?
- Have I summed up my ideas in several sentences within the conclusion?
- Have I included new ideas within the conclusion? If so, remove them.
- Do all of the references used in my essay appear in my reference list?

Referencing your work

Your clinical practice is expected to be based on evidence and facts and the same applies to your academic work. Acknowledging the sources of information used is known as referencing.

Why reference?:
- Shows your understanding of the subject
- Demonstrates how widely you have read
- Indicates the depth of your reading
- Offers support for your views and discussions
- Allows the reader to identify your sources of information in the same way that you will have found references in journal articles and textbooks
- Makes clear to the reader what ideas and information are your own, so you cannot be accused of plagiarism.

When to reference:
- If you use facts, ideas or information from someone else's work:
  - this could be a direct quotation
  - you may have paraphrased them by putting what they said into your own words
  - you may have summarised their work
- Their work could be a journal article, website or in a textbook.

How to reference:

There are a number of systems that are commonly used for referencing, and your own university will have an online tutorial or workshop to guide you through the process. This will tell you exactly how to record the details of the evidence used in your assignment. Different schools within the same university may have slight differences depending on the subject. It's important to get it right as assignment marks are allocated to the accuracy of your referencing.

There are two parts to the process:

- When you indicate the source of your information within your assignment, e.g.:
  - Ward (2020) considers that her clinical experience gained before commencing a nursing associate course was valuable to her development as a trainee nursing associate.
  - Giddings (2020, p. 402) states that "placements gave me a wealth of knowledge into different care environments".
  - Placements can offer insights into different care environments (Giddings, 2020).
- When you create a detailed alphabetical list of all the sources you have referred to, at the end of your assignment. This records the author name, date of the journal, the title of the article, the name of the journal, the volume and part number and finally the page numbers for the article. If the reference is to a book, the author name, date of publication, title of the book, place of publication and the publisher are needed. For website references you need to add the date when the website was accessed.
  - Giddings, S. (2020) Nursing associates... what are they and how does their role fit within the team? *British Journal of Healthcare Assistants*, **14**(8): 400–405.
  - Ward, M. (2020) So you want to be a qualified nursing associate? *British Journal of Healthcare Assistants*, **14**(5): 217–219.

1.6.5 Revising and sitting examinations

The thought of taking an examination creates anxiety in most students. If there is one on your course, don't become overly concerned as exams take many forms.

- Seen exams
  - you know the topics that you will be expected to answer questions about in advance.
- Multiple choice questions (MCQs)
  - you select the answer from several presented to you.
- Open book
  - you have a textbook or key papers to use to answer questions during the exam.
- Short answer
  - you are not required to write essays to answer the questions. Answers may be of varied length indicated by the marks allocated.
- Unseen essay
  - you know the subject, for example communication, but not the questions.

- Objective Structured Clinical Examination (OSCE)
  - OSCEs test your competence in a skill such as taking and recording physiological measurements, usually in a clinical skills laboratory under simulation conditions.
- Practical
  - your clinical practice will be continuously assessed in the clinical area by an experienced assessor. While you are not under typical exam conditions, it is worth remembering that your skills and behaviour are being observed throughout your placements.

Preparing for an examination

Look at past papers

Many past examination papers, usually with the exception of MCQs, are available to read from your university library. They give a flavour of how questions are phrased and popular topics within a subject area. Reading these helps make the unknown more familiar. If past MCQs are not available in your library, there are usually examples on the internet that are good enough for practice.

Revision

Revision is the reinforcing of previous learning, refreshing your memory and understanding. That is why attendance at tutorials and lectures is important, along with good notes. If you didn't learn the topic, you can't revise it and have to start from scratch.

Knowing your preferred learning style will guide you to use posters, diagrams and flashcards or to write out short notes about the topic.
- Start early and allow yourself plenty of time.
- Write a list of topics that you need to revise.
- Allocate two 2-hour revision sessions each day
  - don't try to revise for 2 hours continuously; take short breaks but don't get distracted.
- Create a revision timetable
  - allocate time to specific topics and stick to it. If you overrun in the early part of your timetable it will mean that you cannot revise some of the topics at the end of your list.
- Return to the topic 48 hours, one week and three weeks after you have revised it.
- Don't neglect your diet, exercise and sleep.

Unseen written exams usually require you to write longer answers in a limited amount of time. You must express yourself clearly, keeping to the point. Make sure you stay focused on the question and don't allow yourself to drift away from it.

Know the rules:

- How long is the exam?
- How many questions do I answer?
- Are some questions compulsory?
- Are some questions optional?
- How are marks allocated?
  - is there 100% allocated for the entire answer or are there several sub-sections with different weightings?

In the exam:

During the first ten minutes:

- Read carefully through the questions.
- Decide which ones you will answer and make a note of these.
- Calculate your timings when you should start and finish the questions.

Plan your answer:

- Read the question.
- Underline the verb that tells you how to answer.
- Underline the key ideas and issues.

If the exam question that you had chosen to answer read "Discuss the benefits of effective communication in the nursing associate–patient relationship", you have to answer the question using a discussion. The key issues within the question are 'effective communication' and the 'nursing associate–patient relationship'.

Make sure you:

- Demonstrate an understanding of the subject
- Answer the question as requested, compare, discuss, list and so on.

Study skills are essential to develop competence in your academic work, they reduce the risk of failure and will help you to make the most of any learning opportunities that your course presents (Patidar, 2019).

CHAPTER SUMMARY

- Checking the quality of your study skills and updating deficiencies is a good starting point on your nursing associate course.
- Get into the habit of setting aside regular slots of time to study.
- Ask for support from library staff to find evidence and take advantage of workshops on literature searching and referencing methods.
- Keep the details of all of your sources of evidence safe, save and back up your written assignments frequently.
- Preparing for seminars, tutorials and lectures means that you will learn more from them.

FURTHER READING

Ellis, C. (2020) Passionate about the apprenticeship route. *British Journal of Healthcare Assistants*, **14**(11): 560–562.

Ghisoni, M. and Murphy, P. (eds.) (2019) *Study Skills: for nursing, health and social care*. Lantern Publishing.

Giddings, S. (2020) Nursing associates... what are they and how does their role fit within the team? *British Journal of Healthcare Assistants*, **14**(8): 400–405.

UCAS (2020) *Study Skills Guides*. Available at: https://www.ucas.com/undergraduate/student-life/study-skills-guides (accessed 15 November 2022).

References

NMC (2018) *Standards of Proficiency for Registered Nursing Associates*. Nursing and Midwifery Council. Available at: https://www.nmc.org.uk/standards/standards-for-nursing-associates/standards-of-proficiency-for-nursing-associates or bit.ly/3YcOUZJ (accessed 2 December 2022).

Patidar, J. (2019) Evaluation of study skills in nursing students. *International Journal of Nursing Education*, **11**(3): 26–31.

PROFESSIONAL SKILLS

Linda Bale

This chapter relates directly to outcomes 1.9, 3.4 and 3.5 of the Standards of Proficiency for Nursing Associates (NMC, 2018). However, communication is a fundamental component within the role of the nursing associate and underpins many of the other outcomes that must be achieved for registration with the NMC.

LEARNING OUTCOMES

When you have completed this chapter you should be able to:
- Define communication and identify its importance within the nursing associate role.
- Outline the value of communication in the development of high quality care.
- Describe ways of communicating and how these can be optimised in the clinical environment.
- Discuss factors which may impede communication between patients and the nursing associate.
- Discuss the benefits of team working in the delivery of healthcare and describe the roles and behaviours of team members.
- Identify the stages that teams progress through before becoming fully functioning.
- Explore the similarities and differences between management and leadership, and describe different styles of leadership.

2.1 Introduction

Initially this chapter highlights the importance of communication in the care process, and then describes the ways in which the nursing associate can communicate with patients. It goes on to explore ways of improving communication before identifying factors that inhibit communication within the care environment. The chapter then identifies the value of teamwork and discusses the nature of teams in healthcare. Finally, the characteristics of managers and leaders are described and related to the role of the nursing associate.

2.2 The importance of communication in nursing

The nursing associate is an emerging healthcare professional who will deliver care to individuals of all ages, from different backgrounds and cultures and across all fields of nursing (HEE, 2017; NMC, 2018). The nursing associate proficiency standards (NMC, 2018) indicate that the role has a focus on communication and relationship management skills, emphasising the importance of communication within nursing. All of the proficiencies identified in the standards depend on good communication skills.

Communication was also identified as one of the 6Cs (NHS England, 2015) and described as the key to a good workplace, with benefits for service users and staff alike. The 6Cs are:

- Care
- Compassion
- Courage
- Communication
- Competence
- Commitment.

ACTIVITY 2.1

How important do you think good communication with patients and colleagues is in the delivery of care?

You may have considered some of the following:

- Promotes person-centred care
- Is essential to gain informed consent
- Reduces the risk of errors
- Reduces patients' anxiety
- Allows patients to contribute to their plan of care
- Enriches the therapeutic patient–nurse relationship
- Aids concordance with treatments (concordance is the extent to which a patient follows a prescribed treatment – not only medication – after a discussion and decision-making that includes their values and beliefs)
- Shortens the length of hospital stay
- Promotes good interdisciplinary team working
- Promotes patient safety.

In 2012, the Department of Health (DH, 2012) launched *Compassion in Practice*, a document highlighting the importance of the acquisition of good communication skills by all members of the healthcare team. It viewed these as fundamental to successful compassionate and caring therapeutic relationships between patients and healthcare providers. Furthermore, communication skills are transferable, enhancing the nursing associate's employability skills as well as contributing to the provision of a high standard of person-centred care (NMC, 2018; HEE, 2017; NHS England, 2015).

Building and establishing a professional relationship with patients involves the use of therapeutic communication, an important professional interpersonal process that promotes trust and respect. Therapeutic communication supports the patient identity and helps achieve their health-related goals and outcomes (Arnold and Underman Boggs, 2019; Norman, 2019).

>> **Communication is a fundamental skill for a nursing associate and underpins many of the outcomes that must be achieved for registration with the NMC.**

2.2.1 Defining communication

There are many definitions of communication. In the simplest form it can be defined as the process of transmitting information from one person to another, with a desired response. Wood's (2004) transactional model of communication (see *Figure 2.1*) illustrates the complexities that can arise when two people communicate. Wood identifies that a person's previous experience has an impact on the way information is communicated and on the way that the information is interpreted by the receiver. Factors within individual communicators that may influence the process include their cultural background, language and dialect differences, level of education and the quality of their hearing and vision. The double-headed arrows signify the role each communicator has in decoding

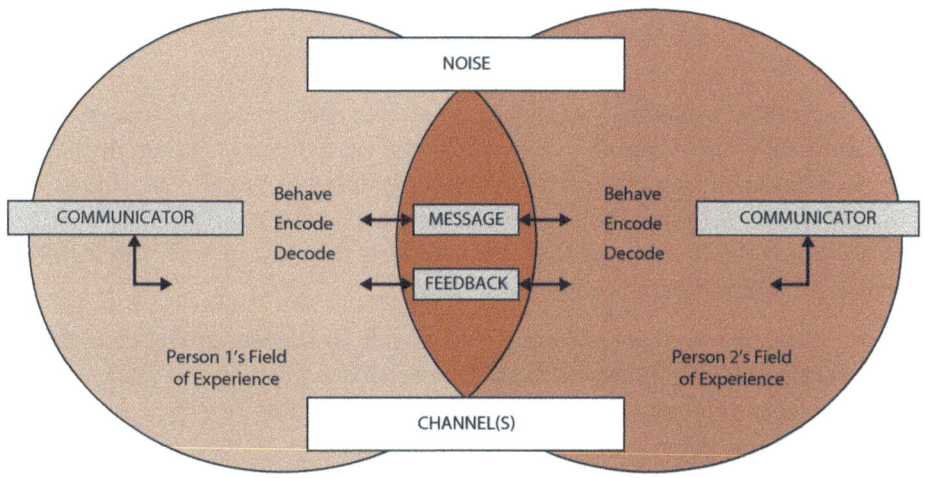

Figure 2.1 *A transactional model of communication. Adapted and modified from Wood (2004).*

the meaning of the communication, and this includes interpreting non-verbal communication such as facial expressions and gestures.

Kennedy-Sheldon (2009) described communication in nursing as the sharing of health-related information between the nurse and the patient, with both involved in the sending and receiving of information. McCabe and Timmins (2013) extend this, describing communication in nursing as interpersonal and as the process of how care and compassion are offered and information, decisions and feelings are shared.

There is debate around whether it is possible to teach undergraduate student nurses the skills required to be good communicators, with some suggesting that such qualities are an inherent attribute within the nurse that can be developed. Freshwater and Stickley (2004) claim that it is necessary for the nurse to have 'emotional intelligence' to develop communication skills and to be able to relate to others.

2.2.2 Types of communication

ACTIVITY 2.2

Think about what the following terms mean to you, and write short notes about your ideas.
- Verbal communication
- Non-verbal communication

Verbal communication

You may have written about this being the spoken word, i.e. what we say during communication.

It is important to remember that language evolves over time and words can have more than one meaning. For example, the word '*tinker*' could imply that someone has been mischievous, as in '*You little tinker*'. It can also be used to describe a process of repairing something, as in 'tinkering'. '*Tinker*' has also been used to refer to someone from the travelling community who travels from place to place repairing items.

The meaning of a word or sentence can be altered by the tone and pitch of the voice. Factors which emphasise the spoken word, like the tone and pitch of the voice and facial expressions, are known as paralinguistics.

ACTIVITY 2.3

Try altering the tone and pitch of your voice when you say the phrase 'meet me at 8pm'.

How many meanings can you achieve from one brief phrase?

You may have conveyed a question, a threat, excitement or worry, but there are several other possibilities.

Non-verbal communication

This is the message that we convey without words through our body language, posture and facial expressions, intentionally or otherwise. Riggio and Feldman (2005) point out that while communication frameworks separate verbal and non-verbal communication, they are intrinsically interlinked.

SOLER is an acronym that has been widely used to enhance nurses' non-verbal communication skills, specifically focusing on the interaction and relationship between the patient and the nurse. This was introduced by Egan (1975) as a strategy to promote 'active listening'. SOLER stands for:

- S – Sit squarely
- O – Open posture
- L – Lean forward
- E – Eye contact
- R – Relax and respond

Stickley (2011) developed the SURETY model, which included the appropriate use of *touch* as part of the communication process. This must be culturally sensitive and relies upon the nurse's intuition.

- S – Sit at an angle to the patient
- U – Uncross legs and arms
- R – Relax
- E – Eye contact
- T – Touch
- Y – Your intuition

The NMC (2018, p. 19) states that nursing associates should 'use appropriate non-verbal communication including touch, eye contact and personal space'. Body language that portrays nurses as rushed, anxious or uncomfortable has been linked to poorer patient outcomes (Riggio and Feldman, 2005).

ACTIVITY 2.4

Try this activity working with a fellow trainee nursing associate. One person acts as the listener and one person shares information.

First: sit with your partner (not using either SOLER or SURETY model) and get them to tell you for a few minutes what they did before they became a trainee nursing associate, then exchange roles.

Secondly: repeat the process using one of the SOLER or SURETY models.

Discuss any differences in the communication process that you noticed. Consider the following: Did the information-giver feel that it was easier to talk when the listener used one of the models? Did it feel like you were being listened to? Did you feel that the listener was interested in what you had to say? Was the communication process enhanced by the use of one of the models?

Remember to try applying one of the models at the next appropriate opportunity on clinical placement.

Written communication

Within healthcare written communication may be in many different formats. It can take the form of an entry into patient records, completing observation charts and compiling referral, transfer and discharge letters. Some records may still need to be handwritten, with others completed digitally, but all records must be clear, contemporary and legible (NMC, 2018).

ACTIVITY 2.5

Spend a few minutes considering the issues that might be encountered if written communication is not clear and legible in the clinical setting.

You may have considered: inappropriate care being given based on illegible assessments (wound care / pressure ulcer management / wrong diet / incorrect equipment for manual handling) and inappropriate referrals made to other healthcare professionals based on illegible observation records. The list is endless and the potential for serious harm very great.

ACTIVITY 2.6

Identify the different types of communication taking place in this scenario:

Kevin is a newly registered nursing associate who is working a morning shift on an adult surgical ward. The shift begins with all team members receiving a

ACTIVITY 2.6 (continued)

structured bedside handover from the night staff. This clinical area prepares a printed or digital copy of the 'handover' information and all team members have access to this.

The nurse who is coordinating the morning shift allocates Kevin a group of patients that he will be caring for that morning. There are patients that need to be prepared for surgery and there will be other patients returning to the ward area post-surgery. A copy of the scheduled theatre list for that day is available for all team members.

During the shift Kevin is kept very busy:
- Answering a telephone call from relatives requiring an update on their family member's condition
- Attending a multidisciplinary team meeting
- Recording vital signs
- Providing support, guidance and feedback / feed forward to a 1st year nursing associate student
- Providing reassurance to a patient who is feeling very anxious prior to their scheduled surgical procedure
- Providing discharge home advice to a patient who has a hearing impairment
- Completing a discharge letter that needs to be emailed to the patient's GP surgery
- Communicating with the community nursing team so that the patient's stitches can be removed on the correct date
- Conducting a handover to the afternoon staff.

2.2.3 Communication and person-centred care

Person-centred care is a term used within healthcare based on the principle of:
- Treating every patient as an individual
- Respecting their choices and decisions as a person
- Ensuring that they have an influence on their care plan and on the delivery of care.

This includes physical, social and psychological considerations.

The Care Act (2014) indicates that all patients should, where possible, be involved in all decisions around their care and support options, and to enable this, the guiding principle must be a person-centred approach. Good communication skills support the delivery of person-centred care.

Person-centred care:
- Promotes dignity and respect
- Reduces patient anxiety

- Promotes patient ability to make informed decisions and consent to treatment options
- Promotes concordance with treatment
- Shortens the length of hospital stay
- Reduces the risk of harm to patients (DH, 2012; PHE, 2018).

Modern healthcare brings many benefits to a wide range of people but it is not without risks, and errors do occur. Improving safety and the quality of care (NMC, 2018) is a national and a global concern and the World Health Organization (WHO, 2017) identifies that delivering safer care in environments that are busy and pressurised is a challenge. It is reported that one in ten hospitalised patients experience harm, with 50% of these identified as being preventable (WHO, 2017). Miscommunication has been documented as the root cause of poorer patient outcomes and safety issues within healthcare (CQC, 2018).

2.2.4 Potential barriers to communication within clinical settings

Barriers exist within the clinical environment that can hinder the communication process. These can be classed as:
- Intrinsic: from within individuals (see *Table 2.1*), or
- Extrinsic: factors in the care environment (see *Table 2.2*).

It can be difficult for a patient to focus on the communication between themselves and members of the healthcare team if they are in pain or feeling

Table 2.1 *Intrinsic factors acting as potential barriers to communication*

Intrinsic factors related to the patient	Intrinsic factors related to you
Language	Language
Culture and religion	Culture and religion
Anxiety	Anxiety around clinical expectations
Previous experience of healthcare	Previous experience/exposure/training
Grief	Values and beliefs
Illness, e.g. aphasia following a stroke	Professional boundaries
Pain	Self-awareness
Sensory impairment	
Cognitive impairment	
Learning difficulty	

worried. If you are feeling anxious, possibly because of limited experience of the clinical situation, this can also have a negative effect on the communication process.

Cultural or language differences between the healthcare team and the patient can also be a barrier to communication, as there may be difficulty understanding the spoken word. Different accents and local dialects can also be a potential barrier.

Sensory impairment can inhibit effective communication. The WHO (2017) defines this as when one of the senses no longer functions at normal capacity – sight, hearing, taste, touch, smell and/or spatial awareness. Hearing loss is projected to be among the top ten causes of burden of disease by 2030, and age-related visual impairment is also predicted to move up the burden of disease ranking, placing additional demands on the communication skills of nursing associates.

It is recognised that within healthcare, staff do not consistently adapt appropriately the way they communicate with people who have a hearing impairment. Healthcare providers often lack understanding of the barrier that this creates in actively engaging these individuals with healthcare services (Middleton *et al.*, 2010). An additional obstacle to consider since the Covid-19 pandemic is the need for healthcare staff to wear personal protective equipment (PPE) including a face mask, which may impede clarity of speech and hinder an individual's ability to lip-read.

There is evidence that the physical layout of hospital wards affects the quality of communication. When hospitalised, patients are placed in unfamiliar environments with little or no control of their surroundings. They are reliant

Table 2.2 *Extrinsic factors acting as potential barriers to communication*

Extrinsic factors that may affect the patient	Extrinsic factors that may affect you
The environment	The environment
Language – medical jargon and abbreviations	Time
Lack of access to communication tools	Access to training
Lack of continuity in healthcare personnel allocation	Patient allocation and work-load
Privacy	
Unequal power relationships	

on the healthcare team for information and care (Tindle *et al.*, 2020). Many healthcare settings are busy and noisy, and it can be a challenge to create an environment that is conducive to good communication. Healthcare staff may become familiar with this environment and can fail to recognise it as a barrier to effective communication (Ali, 2018), but the nursing associate is held to be professionally accountable by the NMC and expected to create an environment that upholds patient confidentiality and privacy (NMC, 2018).

It is widely recognised that adapting language to suit each individual patient and situation is essential (Pitt and Hendrickson, 2019), but the use of medical jargon within healthcare can create a barrier, giving the patient a feeling of an unequal power relationship.

There are concerns over the workload of nurses (Kwame and Petrucka, 2021) and the number of patients allocated to each nurse on a shift. Workload influences the time a nurse has to communicate with each patient and appearing to be very busy may deter patients from interacting with nurses. You will be sharing some of the nurses' clinical workload so remember to take every opportunity to communicate with patients and try not to look too busy all of the time, even if you are.

ACTIVITY 2.7

Consider the environments below and list potential environmental barriers that may hinder communication:
- Hospital inpatient ward
- Hospital outpatient department
- GP practice
- Patient's own home
- Care home
- Day centre.

The NMC (2018) indicates that part of being an accountable professional nursing associate includes the responsibility of communicating effectively and compassionately with every patient and with any carers or family members. The DH (2012) guidance *Compassion in Practice* identifies six fundamental elements that support delivery in practice on a culture of caring, compassion and consideration in nursing. Effective communication is one of these six fundamental elements. Having discussed the importance of effective communication, it is essential to acknowledge that successful communication is a vital component for the establishment of both productive team working and leadership skills.

RECAP

- Effective communication is fundamental to healthcare and is one of the 6Cs.
- Verbal communication is the spoken word. The meanings of words can change over time, and the pitch and tone of your voice can also convey different meanings.
- The message that we convey without words through our body language, posture and facial expressions is known as non-verbal communication.
- Written communication is important in keeping patient records, completing observation charts and compiling referral, transfer and discharge letters, and it must be clear and legible.

2.3 Team working and leadership

Over a decade on, the assertion by Reeves *et al.* (2011) that successful team working is a near-universal aspiration throughout the health and social care sector remains as true as ever. Being described as a member of the nursing team by the NMC, the nursing associate role has been developed to play an important part in the team, bridging the gap between healthcare assistants and registered nurses. As such, a nursing associate will not only be working with colleagues who occupy the same role, but will also collaborate and work closely with other healthcare professionals. As team working is an essential characteristic of the nursing associate role, having an awareness of successful team working is important.

Although varying definitions exist, it can be argued that the essential characteristics of a team include being a collective group of people who interact with each other in order to achieve shared goals. As such, as Gopee and Galloway (2017) argue, a team can be defined as a group of individuals who work

>> **Nursing associates bridge the gap between healthcare assistants and registered nurses and also work with other colleagues as part of a healthcare team.**

together in order to deliver an organisation's services based upon shared aims and objectives, and who, both as individuals and collectively, feel accountable for the achievement of an organisation's aims. Breaking the concept of a team down into its component parts, Benson (2010) argues that a team can be described thus:

- A set of people engaged in frequent interactions
- They identify with one another
- They are defined by others as a group
- They share beliefs, values and norms about areas of common interest
- They define themselves as a group
- They come together to work on common tasks and for agreed purposes.

ACTIVITY 2.8

Think about the teams that you are in or have been part of. These could be sporting, musical, leisure or work-related.

What teams have you been a member of?

What matters most to you about being in a team?

There are five different types of teams found within a healthcare setting:

1. Core teams – team leaders and members who are directly involved in the delivery of patient care, including nurses, doctors, dentists, etc., as well as the patient themselves and carers.
2. Coordinating teams – teams responsible for the day-to-day management and coordination of core teams.
3. Contingency teams – these are those teams which are drawn together in light of a specific or emergent event, such as a cardiac arrest, disaster relief teams, or rapid response teams.
4. Ancillary teams – consisting of individuals whose actions are task-specific but who have limited involvement with patient care, such as cleaners and domestic staff.
5. Support services and administration – individuals who provide task-specific indirect services, as well as executive leaders who have 24-hour accountability for an organisation.

From this list of teams, the nursing associate, working with other nursing associates, would be categorised as a member of a core team.

2.3.1 Benefits of team working

Effective team working contributes significantly to improved outcomes and higher quality care (HEE, 2021) and is considered a vital prerequisite for good practice (Gopee and Galloway, 2017). For West (2012), a well-organised and structured team of health professionals contributes to improved patient mortality and morbidity, while reducing the number of staff absences. Additionally, Rosen *et al.* (2018) argue that for healthcare professionals, working in an effective team can enhance a professional's existing skill set and encourage them to develop new skills. Moreover, Borrill *et al.* (2000) asserted that professionals who regularly worked closely in a team reported lower levels of stress compared to those who spent less time in a team. Consequently, as Gopee and Galloway (2017) contend, positive outcomes from working in a team include increased job satisfaction, reduced staff turnover, professional innovation, and improved patient outcomes.

2.3.2 Interdisciplinary team working

Healthcare teams bring together health professionals with different skills and expertise who can work together to provide the best possible care and support for patients. Within the literature, and among professionals themselves, various terms are used to describe this process, such as multidisciplinary, multiprofessional, transdisciplinary, interdisciplinary and interprofessional. As Choi and Pak (2006) argue, such terms are frequently used inconsistently and interchangeably, leading to confusion. While attempts have been made to identify specific definitions, they all broadly have in common the notion of professionals from different disciplinary and professional backgrounds coming together, combining their skills and knowledge, to achieve the same goals and outcomes. For the purpose of clarity, here the term interdisciplinary will be used.

With nursing associates working closely with both healthcare assistants and registered nurses, interdisciplinary team working defines the nursing associate role. For Nancarrow *et al.* (2013), the need for interdisciplinary team working has become ever more necessary for such reasons as the following:

1. An ageing population has meant an increasing number of patients with complex conditions and comorbidities associated with chronic illness.
2. The increasing complexity of skills and knowledge required to meet the needs of service users.
3. Increasing specialisation among healthcare professionals, meaning that no single professional can meet the complex needs of patients.
4. Greater policy focus among governments which encourages the process.
5. It aids the process of quality improvement.

Many of these reasons have been instrumental in the growth and development of the nursing associate role, with reasons two and three in the list above being of particular importance.

For an interdisciplinary team to be successful, Nancarrow *et al.* (2013) identify ten characteristics:

1. Good communication
2. Respecting and understanding roles
3. Appropriate skill mix
4. Quality and outcomes of care
5. Appropriate team processes and resources
6. Clear vision
7. Flexibility of the team and those who are part of it
8. Leadership and management
9. Positive relationships between members and support
10. Training and development.

While a number of these characteristics pertain to the team as a whole, as an individual nursing associate within a wider team of professionals, it is important that you:

- Display good communication
- Have an awareness and understanding of your role and those of others
- Put into practice effectively your own skills
- Have a clear understanding of the aims and objectives of the team
- Develop positive relationships with all members including other nursing associates as well as other professionals
- Ensure that you continually engage in the process of professional development.

Patients are unlikely to be cared for by one healthcare professional, and effective team working has the additional benefit of improving patient safety and outcomes. In preparation for future roles, it is recommended that all healthcare students begin using the principles of teamwork and collaboration to enable them to become competent members of an interprofessional team (WHO, 2010).

The nursing associate needs to be aware of human factors that can influence the way a team functions. These include an individual's behaviour and characteristics. Becoming aware of our own strengths and weaknesses, a conscious process of self-awareness in which we develop an understanding of ourselves (Rawlinson, 1990), is essential when working in a caring environment, as it is necessary to question the effect we have on others within the team (Burnard, 1992). This in turn helps us to relate to other people, an essential role of the nursing associate who is expected to demonstrate relationship management skills at the point of registration (NMC, 2018).

ACTIVITY 2.9

List the teams that nurses and nursing associates work within.

List the members of teams that you are part of, e.g. healthcare support worker, speech therapist.

2.3.3 Team roles and development

Looking closely at specific teams, in order for any team to function as a whole, it is important that individuals are engaged in roles and tasks which are suited to them. Belbin's (1997) theory about how teams function can explain the strengths and weaknesses of a team and is frequently used to prepare individuals for their team roles. A 'self-perception inventory' can be completed by individuals to establish their preferred way of working within a team. Belbin identified nine individual behaviours that contribute to the functioning of a team. He categorised these into three broad areas: action-oriented, people-oriented and thought-oriented. This doesn't mean that there have to be

Table 2.3 *Belbin's team roles*

Action-oriented roles		People-oriented roles		Thought-oriented roles	
Who they are	**What they do**	**Who they are**	**What they do**	**Who they are**	**What they do**
Shaper	Challenges the team to improve	Coordinator	Acts as a chairperson	Plant	Presents new ideas and approaches
Implementer	Puts ideas into action	Team worker	Encourages cooperation	Monitor Evaluator	Analyses the options
Completer Finisher	Makes sure things get done on time	Resource Investigator	Explores outside opportunities	Specialist	Provides specialised skills

nine people in every team. Most team members will play more than one role and this can change over time.

The advantages of knowing about the roles and associated behaviours of team members are that:

- It provides the opportunity to create a more balanced team by getting the right people to perform the right job.
- The strengths of individual team members can be developed.
- Individual weaknesses can be managed.
- The self-awareness of team members is increased, which can lead to improved contributions by team members.

ACTIVITY 2.10

Look up Belbin's theory and complete the questionnaire to see what sort of role you would play as a team member (www.belbin.com/about/belbin-team-roles).

ACTIVITY 2.11

Think about the teams that you have been part of. These could be sporting, musical, leisure or work-related. What factors stopped the team(s) working as well as they could have done?

You may have experienced some of the following: personality clashes between team members, poor communication, rivalry and/or conflict between team members, dominating team members, team members not pulling their weight, unclear team goals and some team members having too great an influence on decisions.

Tuckman (1965) developed a theory of team development proposing that every team moves between four stages: forming, storming, norming and performing (see *Figure 2.2*). The performing stage of this process is the most productive. Tuckman's theory (1965) is still relevant today, as newly formed healthcare teams have to develop to function effectively, going through the stages proposed by Tuckman, irrespective of the timescale they are given. An appreciation of the Tuckman theory can help individuals to gain an understanding of the characteristics of an effective team, and this can support members of a team to develop mutual respect and good cohesion (Mickan and Rodger, 2005).

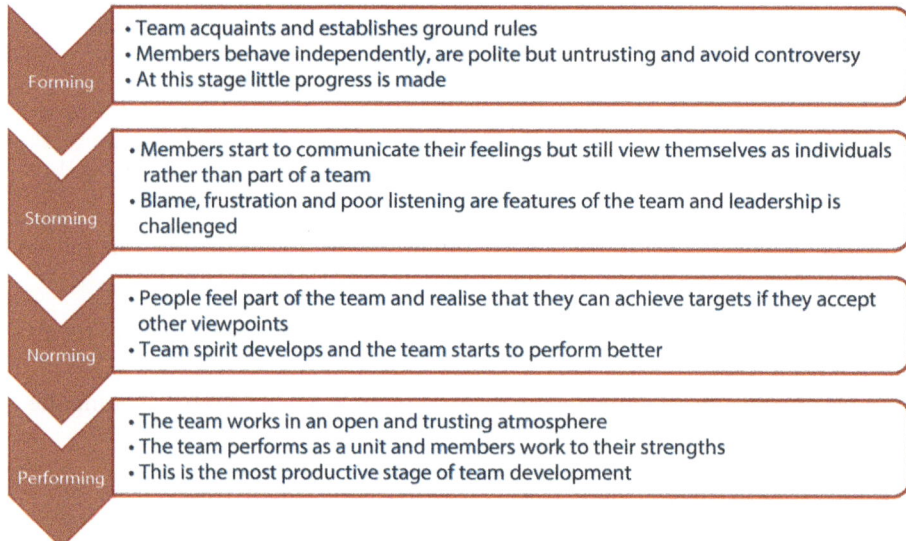

Forming
- Team acquaints and establishes ground rules
- Members behave independently, are polite but untrusting and avoid controversy
- At this stage little progress is made

Storming
- Members start to communicate their feelings but still view themselves as individuals rather than part of a team
- Blame, frustration and poor listening are features of the team and leadership is challenged

Norming
- People feel part of the team and realise that they can achieve targets if they accept other viewpoints
- Team spirit develops and the team starts to perform better

Performing
- The team works in an open and trusting atmosphere
- The team performs as a unit and members work to their strengths
- This is the most productive stage of team development

Figure 2.2 *Tuckman's stages of group development, from Craig and Mckeown (2015).*

ACTIVITY 2.12

Review the categories in *Figure 2.2* and think about your membership of a current team. Can you identify what stage your team is in?

Once the healthcare team has been formed, it will continue to evolve and work with other healthcare teams to provide high standard person-centred care to patients. This is a common goal for all the healthcare providers within a team. The NMC (2018) requires the nursing associate to be aware of the role and responsibilities of the different members of the multidisciplinary team and to work effectively as part of this team.

There can be barriers to effective team working in the clinical environment (see *Table 2.4*).

Table 2.4 *The five dysfunctions of a team (Lencioni, 2002)*

Inattention to results	The pursuit of individual goals and personal status erodes the focus on collective success
Avoidance of account-ability	The need to avoid interpersonal discomfort prevents team members from holding one another accountable
Lack of commitment	The lack of clarity or buy-in prevents team members from making decisions they will stick to
Fear of conflict	The desire to preserve artificial harmony stifles the occurrence of productive ideological conflict
Absence of trust	The fear of being vulnerable with team members prevents the building of trust within the team

There can be barriers to effective team working in the clinical environment, and miscommunication (both verbal and written) between all members of the multidisciplinary team has been associated with patient safety incidents and poor patient outcomes (WHO, 2007).

2.4 Leadership and management

The NHS Leadership Academy (2015) identifies the need for the NHS to develop leadership capabilities within all members of the healthcare team to ensure that the care services provided continue to improve. The Academy states that leadership can be learnt by everyone, and leadership behaviours are applicable to all staff at all levels and are not specific to a job role or grade.

First, it would be helpful to define what leadership is.

The NHS Leadership Academy (2015) defines this simply as "the art of motivating a group of people to act towards achieving a common goal". Good leadership skills are connected to improved patient care and patient outcomes and to staff wellbeing. The King's Fund (2015) identifies the importance of leaders in the NHS, as they are critical in shaping organisational culture. A culture where staff can question without fear, feel empowered and share learning through teamwork is known to enhance the quality of care provided.

The NMC (2018) nursing associate proficiencies identify the standards required of the emerging nursing associate, and these include having the awareness of policy and political drivers that impact on health and care provision, and the requirement to contribute to team reflective activities and review of the quality of care provided. Nursing associates have a professional duty of care to provide feedback on the care delivered by others and to review the quality of care provided.

It is important for nursing associates to have an appreciation of the different leadership models and how these apply to their own clinical and professional development. HEE (2018) recognises the value of developing leadership skills in pre-registration healthcare programmes.

The terms 'manager' and 'leader' are often used interchangeably and sometimes appear to be interchangeable, and indeed a manager may also have a leadership role and a leader may have a management role. However, for the continued development of healthcare services it is widely recognised that the two roles need to be distinguished (Jones and Bennett, 2018).

ACTIVITY 2.13

Think about the leaders and managers (healthcare, sporting, political, or from any other field) that you have worked with or are aware of. Write down what you consider to be the differences between a manager and a leader.

A manager can be described as someone who ensures that processes are in place in order that tasks are completed within agreed timeframes. Planning, controlling people and organising is a key part of their role. Rigolosi (2012) identifies the manager's role as one that is often appointed or elected to the authoritarian position and holds the responsibility of achieving identified organisational goals.

A leader does not have to hold management responsibilities and does not have to be elected or appointed. Many people take on the role of a leader without their role being clearly established or defined. Belbin (1997) suggests that leadership is quite often not part of the job role but is a quality that can be brought to a job role.

A good nurse leader has been described as someone who can inspire others to work towards a common goal. Within healthcare this would quite often refer to patient care, patient experiences, and patient satisfaction and outcomes. A leader is responsible for the outcomes. It is widely recognised that an effective nurse leader holds a set of distinctive qualities and they have been described as role models.

Organisations like the NHS need both managers and leaders.

ACTIVITY 2.14

Think about times when you have acted as a leader of any team. Make a note of what made you stand out as the leader and how you led the team.

Thinking back to leaders you have worked with, what made them a good leader?

As early as 1978 two models of leadership were described by Burns (1978). These were:

- Transformational – leaders motivate followers, develop a shared sense of ownership and shared goals
- Transactional – often described as the model where benefits (rewards) are supplied for performance and achievement.

There are five key leadership styles that require some definition:

- **Bureaucratic:** this type of leadership style ensures all rules, policies and procedures are followed in a strict order and does not encourage questioning or ideas from the team members.
- **Autocratic:** all decisions are made by the leader and all control is maintained by that leader. There is little or no input from team members around planning or decision-making.
- **Democratic:** planning and decisions are made collectively as a team. All team members are encouraged to provide input and ideas are shared and encouraged.
- **Charismatic:** this leader will be self-confident and have a powerful personality. They will be excellent communicators that are compassionate and determined to reach the set goals and objectives.
- **Laissez-faire:** this leadership style allows the team members to plan and organise themselves with little or no input from the leader. This leader trusts the team members to achieve the goal.

ACTIVITY 2.15

Review the five leadership styles and write down two advantages and two disadvantages for each style.

Which style of leadership is most similar to your own?

The NHS Leadership Academy (2015) identifies the importance of personal qualities within nursing leadership, such as self-awareness and having the ability to be aware of one's own strengths and abilities. It is recognised that the behaviour of the leader affects the behaviour of others within that team.

The NHS Leadership Academy (2015) identifies nine dimensions of leadership behaviour.

These are:

- Inspiring a shared purpose
- Leading with care
- Evaluating information
- Connecting our service
- Sharing the vision
- Engaging the team

- Holding to account
- Developing capability
- Influencing for results.

Access www.leadershipacademy.nhs.uk for further reading and information.

Leadership does not necessarily need to be undertaken as a formal process and the nursing associate may have many qualities that naturally lend themselves to leading a team of colleagues. Indeed the Chartered Institute of Professional Development (CIPD) sees leadership as "the capacity to influence people by means of personal attributes and/or behaviours, to achieve a common goal".

ACTIVITY 2.16: CASE STUDY

Prior to starting nursing associate training, Kevin gained considerable care experience supporting young adults with a learning disability. Because of this experience, the registered members of the nursing team and students looked to Kevin for guidance in how best they might support a patient with a learning disability in their clinical setting.

Write down what personal qualities are required by Kevin to assist him in sharing his experiences with other team members.

The NMC (2018) nursing associate standards of proficiency identify the importance of working in teams and improving the quality of care to the nursing associate's development as an accountable practitioner. This in turn aligns to informal and formal nursing associate leadership within healthcare and all nursing associates have a responsibility to ensure that they familiarise themselves with leadership models. The WHO (2020) identifies the importance of investment in the emerging workforce, and this is to include leadership programmes to nurture leadership development in aspiring nurses and nursing associates.

CHAPTER SUMMARY

- Communication underpins all activities in the nursing associate role. Understanding factors that may inhibit communication as well as how to improve your communication is a prerequisite to high quality care.
- Nursing associates are part of larger healthcare teams. The effectiveness of a team improves over a period of time and depends on having the appropriate mix of people and professionals. Effective team working delivers benefits for patients and team members.
- Managers fulfil an important role ensuring that care-related work is completed in a timely manner and to agreed care standards.
- Leadership is important as it is motivational to staff and enhances patient care and satisfaction.

FURTHER READING

Communication

Barber, C. (2016) Communication and the 6Cs: the patient experience. Available at: www.nursingtimes.net/roles/hospital-nurses/communication-and-the-6cs-the-patient-experience-30-05-2016 or bit.ly/43871nl (accessed 2 December 2022).

Bruton, J., Norton, C., Smyth, N., Ward, H. and Day, S. (2016) Nurse handover: patient and staff experiences. *British Journal of Nursing*, **25(7)**: 386–393.

Norman, K. (2019) *Communication Skills*. Lantern Publishing.

Pavord, E. and Donnelly, E. (2015) *Communication and Interpersonal Skills*. Lantern Publishing.

Teamwork

Nancarrow, S., Booth, A., Ariss, S. *et al.* (2013) Ten principles of good interdisciplinary team work. *Human Resources for Health*, **11(19)**.

Robson, R. (2016) Tools and techniques to improve teamwork and avoid patient harm. *Nursing Times*. Available at: www.nursingtimes.net/clinical-archive/patient-safety/tools-and-techniques-to-improve-teamwork-and-avoid-patient-harm-12-12-2016 or bit.ly/3kCMxS8 (accessed 2 December 2022).

Rosen, M.A., DiazGranados, D., Dietz, A.S. *et al.* (2018) Teamwork in healthcare: key discoveries enabling safer, high-quality care. *American Psychologist*, **73(4)**: 433–450.

Leadership

Jebb, P. (2021) Wherever there are leaders, there must be followers. Available at: www.rcn.org.uk/magazines/career/2021/june/wherever-there-are-leaders-there-must-be-followers or bit.ly/3kCMX1c (accessed 2 December 2022).

Jones, L. and Bennett, C.L. (2018) *Leadership: for nursing, health and social care students*. Lantern Publishing.

References

Ali, M. (2018) Communication skills 2: overcoming barriers to effective communication. *Nursing Times*, **114**(1): 40–42.

Arnold, C. and Underman Boggs, A. (2019) *Professional Communication Skills for Nurses*. Elsevier.

Belbin, M. (1997) *Changing the Way we Work*. Butterworth-Heinemann.

Benson, J. (2010) *Working More Creatively with Groups*. Routledge.

Borrill, C., West, M., Shapiro, D. and Rees, A. (2000) Team working and effectiveness in health care. *British Journal of Healthcare Management*, **6**(8): 364–371.

Burnard, P. (1992) *Know Yourself! Self-Awareness Activities for Nurses*. Scutari.

Burns, J. (1978) *Leadership*. Harper & Row.

Care Act (2014) Available at: www.legislation.gov.uk/ukpga/2014/23/contents/enacted (accessed 2 December 2022).

Choi, B.C. and Pak, A.W. (2006) Multidisciplinarity, interdisciplinarity and transdisciplinarity in health research, services, education and policy: 1. Definitions, objectives, and evidence of effectiveness. *Clin Invest Med*, **29**(6): 351–64.

CQC (2018) *State of Care*. Care Quality Commission. Available at: www.cqc.org.uk/news/stories/state-care-201718-published or bit.ly/3SAKACp (accessed 2 December 2022).

Craig, M. and Mckeown, D. (2015) Teambuilding 1: How to build effective teams in healthcare. *Nursing Times*; **111**(14): 16–18.

DH (2012) *Compassion in practice.* Department of Health. Available at: www.england.nhs.uk/wp-content/uploads/2012/12/compassion-in-practice.pdf or bit.ly/3Zw1ggt (accessed 2 December 2022).

Egan, G. (1975) *The Skilled Helper: a systematic approach to effective helping.* Brooks Cole.

Freshwater, D. and Stickley, T. (2004) The heart of the art: emotional intelligence in nurse education. *Nursing Inquiry,* **11**(2): 91–99.

Gopee, N. and Galloway, J. (2017) *Leadership and Management in Healthcare,* 3rd edition. Sage.

HEE (2017) *Trainee Nursing Associate Programme.* Health Education England. Available at: www.hee.nhs.uk/our-work/nursing-associates/trainee-nursing-associate-programme or bit.ly/3ZxfBcK (accessed 2 December 2022).

HEE (2018) *Maximising Leadership Learning in the Pre-Registration Healthcare Curricula.* Health Education England. Available at: www.hee.nhs.uk/sites/default/files/documents/Guidelines%20-%20Maximising%20Leadership%20in%20the%20Pre-reg%20Healthcare%20Curricula_0.pdf or bit.ly/3YfPdmq (accessed 22 December 2022).

HEE (2021) *Working Differently Together: progressing a one workforce approach.* Health Education England. Available at: www.hee.nhs.uk/sites/default/files/documents/HEE_MDT_Toolkit_V1.1.pdf or bit.ly/3ZsfgYD (accessed 22 December 2022).

Jones, L. and Bennett, C.L. (2018) *Leadership: for nursing, health and social care students.* Lantern Publishing.

Kennedy-Sheldon, L. (2009) *Communication for Nurses: talking with patients.* Jones & Bartlett Learning.

Kwame, A. and Petrucka, P.M. (2021) A literature-based study of patient-centered care and communication in nurse-patient interactions: barriers, facilitators, and the way forward. *BMC Nursing,* **20** (158). Available at: https://bmcnurs.biomedcentral.com/articles/10.1186/s12912-021-00684-2 or bit.ly/3kEjjCg (accessed 9 January 2023).

Lencioni, P. (2002) *The Five Dysfunctions of a Team.* Jossey-Bass.

McCabe, C. and Timmins, F. (2013) *Communication Skills for Nursing Practice.* Palgrave Macmillan.

Mickan, S.M. and Rodger, S.A. (2005) Effective health care teams: a model of six characteristics developed from shared perceptions. *J Interprof Care,* **19**(4): 358–70.

Middleton, A., Niruban, A., Girling, G. and Myint, P.K. (2010) Communicating in a healthcare setting with people who have hearing loss. *BMJ,* 341: c4672. Available at: www.academia.edu/7085820/Communicating_in_a_healthcare_setting_with_people_who_have_hearing_loss or bit.ly/3KMDSal (accessed 2 December 2022).

Nancarrow, S., Booth, A., Ariss, S. *et al.* (2013) Ten principles of good interdisciplinary team work. *Human Resources for Health,* **11(19).** Available at: https://human-resources-health.biomedcentral.com/articles/10.1186/1478-4491-11-19#citeas or bit.ly/3J3N9K3 (accessed 2 December 2022).

NHS England (2015*)* Introducing the 6Cs. Available at: www.england.nhs.uk/6cs/wp-content/uploads/sites/25/2015/03/introducing-the-6cs.pdf or bit.ly/3ZxykEG (accessed 2 December 2022).

NHS Leadership Academy (2015) Developing better leaders, delivering better care.

NMC (2018) *Standards of Proficiency for Registered Nursing Associates.* Nursing and Midwifery Council. Available at: www.nmc.org.uk/standards/standards-for-nursing-associates or bit.ly/3SBoYFT (accessed 2 December 2022).

Norman, K. (2019) *Communication Skills: for nursing and healthcare students.* Lantern Publishing.

Pitt, M. and Hendrickson, M. (2019) Eradicating jargon–oblivion – a proposed classification system of medical jargon. *Journal of General Internal Medicine,* **35**(6): 1861–1864.

Public Health England (PHE) (2018) *Health Profile for England: 2018.* Available at: www.gov.uk/government/publications/health-profile-for-england-2018 (accessed 2 December 2022).

Rawlinson, J. (1990) Self-awareness: conceptual influences, contribution to nursing, and approaches to attainment. *Nurse Education Today,* **10**(2): 111–117.

Reeves, S., Goldman, J., Gilbert, J. *et al.* (2011) A scoping review to improve conceptual clarity of interprofessional interventions. *Journal of Interprofessional Care,* **25**(3): 167–174.

Riggio, E. and Feldman, R. (2005) *Applications of Nonverbal Communication*. Taylor & Francis Group.

Rigolosi, E. (2012) *Management and Leadership in Nursing and Health Care: an experiential approach*, 3rd edition. Springer Publishing Company.

Rosen, M.A., DiazGranados, D., Dietz, A.S. *et al.* (2018) Teamwork in healthcare: key discoveries enabling safer, high-quality care. *American Psychologist,* **73**(4): 433–450.

Stickley, T. (2011) From SOLER to SURETY for effective non-verbal communication. *Nurse Education in Practice,* **11**(6): 395–398.

The King's Fund (2015) *Leadership and Leadership Development in Health Care: the evidence base.* Available at: www.kingsfund.org.uk/publications/leadership-and-leadership-development-health-care or bit.ly/3mgAScc (accessed 2 December 2022).

Tindle, K., David, A., Carlisle, S. *et al.* (2020) Relationship of the built environment on nursing communication patterns in the emergency department: a task performance and analysis time study. *Journal of Emergency Nursing,* **46**(40): 440–448.

Tuckman, B.W. (1965) Developmental sequence in small groups. *Psychological Bulletin,* **63**(6): 384–399.

West, M.A. (2012) *Effective Teamwork: practical lessons from organizational research.* Wiley.

WHO (2007) *Communication During Patient Hand-Overs.* Available at: https://cdn.who.int/media/docs/default-source/integrated-health-services-(ihs)/psf/patient-safety-solutions/ps-solution3-communication-during-patient-handovers.pdf?sfvrsn=7a54c664_4&ua=1 or bit.ly/3IDtDmg (accessed 2 December 2022).

WHO (2010) *Framework for Action on Interprofessional Education & Collaborative Practice.* Available at: http://apps.who.int/iris/bitstream/handle/10665/70185/WHO_HRH_HPN_10.3_eng.pdf?sequence=1 or bit.ly/41zqcW6 (accessed 2 December 2022).

WHO (2017) *Patient Safety: making health care safer.* Available at: https://apps.who.int/iris/bitstream/handle/10665/255507/WHO-HIS-SDS-2017.11-eng.pdf;jsessionid=E8EBB88531820DD7FE00BA236DAF7B99?sequence=1 or bit.ly/3EMitKx (accessed 2 December 2022).

WHO (2020) *State of the World's Nursing.* Available at: www.who.int/publications/i/item/9789240003279 (accessed 2 December 2022).

Wood, J. (2004) *Communication Theories in Action: an introduction.* Thompson Learning.

VALUES AND ETHICS

Anneyce Knight and Nevin Mehmet

This chapter relates to outcomes 1.1, 1.2, 1.3 and 1.11 within the
***Standards of Proficiency for Nursing Associates* (NMC, 2018b).**

LEARNING OUTCOMES

When you have completed this chapter you should be able to:
- Understand what personal and professional values are.
- Briefly describe the ethical theories of utilitarianism, deontology and virtue ethics.
- Explain the 'four principles' of autonomy, beneficence, non-maleficence and justice.
- Demonstrate an understanding of the importance of values and ethics and how they apply to your everyday practice as a nursing associate.
- Define accountability and develop an awareness of who you are accountable to.

3.1 Introduction

This chapter begins by explaining what values and ethics are and why they are important to you, both as a trainee nursing associate and later as a registered nursing associate. The chapter outlines the ethical theories of utilitarianism, deontology and virtue ethics. It then moves on to explain and discuss Beauchamp and Childress' (2019) four ethical principles, namely autonomy, beneficence, non-maleficence and justice, and considers how they relate to your everyday practice. The chapter concludes with a discussion on the importance of accountability within your role.

By the end of this chapter there is an expectation that you will have explored and gained some understanding of your personal values as well as enhanced your knowledge of the professional values and ethics that underpin your daily nursing practice. These are embedded within the Nursing and Midwifery

Council (NMC) (2018a) *The Code: professional standards of practice and behaviour for nurses, midwives and nursing associates* (henceforth NMC *Code*), the NMC (2018b) *Standards of Proficiency for Nursing Associates* (henceforth NMC *Standards*) and the 6Cs (DH, 2012). The 6Cs are:

- Care
- Compassion
- Courage
- Communication
- Competence
- Commitment.

3.2 What are values and ethics?

3.2.1 Values

The Oxford English Dictionary (2010) talks about values as being things we desire and that are of use or of importance to us. In a sense, values can be regarded as particular types of beliefs or goals about what we regard as worthy. This provides a basis for our decision-making about what is considered to be right and wrong. Much philosophical writing has centred on the possible sources of values, which include family, friends, education, society, religion and culture. Religion (of whatever particular kind or viewpoint) and family are considered the strongest and most influential sources; nevertheless, all these sources are powerful in shaping an individual's likes, dislikes, perspectives, prejudices and judgements that can shape our behaviours (Halstead and Reiss, 2003; Duncan, 2010).

Dworkin (1995) developed a useful account of values and their nature by arguing that there are three kinds of values: subjective, instrumental and intrinsic. Subjective values are those that relate to our preferences or strong likes/dislikes and tend to centre around our desires. Instrumental values are those that may be of use. Intrinsic values are much harder to define and it is often impossible to identify a definitive set of core intrinsic values. These values frequently cannot be reduced to a preference or usefulness, for instance, when applied to things that are essential to being human. One example would be social justice, which is concerned with the distribution of factors such as wealth and opportunities within society.

Understanding your own personal values, and how you are motivated and driven by your own core values, is important for your professional nursing practice. Although the form, nature and sources of values are uncertain, and often disputed among philosophers due to their complexity, it is important to recognise that our values may differ between us. In healthcare disagreements about what may be important, or what should be done and how, often occur. If healthcare is about creating better lives (or at least making the conditions of living and dying more tolerable) then there is a need to know what motivates us in our work, and why we take the decisions and act in the ways that we do to support our clinical decision-making (Duncan, 2010). The knowledge and understanding of your own personal values will support you in your role as nursing associates in distinguishing between personal and professional values.

Professional values are a set of standards that are favoured by experts and professional groups as a way of establishing frameworks for setting and evaluating behaviours (Poorchangizi *et al.*, 2019). The fundamental

>> **Core professional values are often embedded in ethical codes such as the NMC *Code*.**

professional nursing values are human dignity, equality among patients and prevention of suffering (Rassin, 2008), as well as integrity, altruism and honesty (NMC, 2018a; Poorchangizi *et al.*, 2019). Duncan (2010) claims that everyone involved in healthcare should have a fundamental concern with values *and* ethics and often core professional values are embedded within ethical codes, such as the NMC (2018a) *Code* which you must abide by.

3.2.2 Ethics

Ethics is a branch of philosophy that addresses questions about morality. Therefore, when ethics is used in the context of moral philosophy, it is often concerned with the study of morality, moral problems and moral judgements which are involved in clinical decision-making. Ethics attempts to define what is good, evil (bad), right and wrong (Mehmet, 2011).

Philosophers have contributed to three main ethical theories: utilitarianism, deontology and virtue ethics.

Utilitarianism is the consequence-based theory of Jeremy Bentham (1748–1832) and John Stuart Mill (1806–73) which centres on the idea that an action is morally good if it produces the greatest amount of good (greater good for the greater number).

Deontology (from the Greek word *deon*, meaning duty) is the normative ethical theory according to Immanuel Kant (1734–1804) who proposed that the morality of an action should be based on whether that action itself is right or wrong under a set of moral rules, rather than based on the consequences of the action.

Virtue ethics is a moral theory that focuses on the character of the individual, which is the moral concern, and someone who shows virtues such as kindness and generosity is the model of moral conduct (see *Section 3.4*). These ethical theories are general ways of thinking and display the richness of moral reasoning. However, it is not always appropriate to adopt one theory and apply it in all situations, as none covers all moral eventualities.

In addition to the ethical theories to support decision-making in practice, Beauchamp and Childress (2019) considered deontology as the foundation for developing a simpler and more effective way of supporting ethical dilemmas/ issues and situations. They developed an ethical framework with four principles; autonomy, beneficence, non-maleficence and justice (see *Section 3.5*).

It is important to note that the terms 'values' and 'ethics' are often used interchangeably. Though the two are different, ethics are often embedded within professional codes, such as the NMC (2018a) *Code*. This enables us to consider what may be right or wrong in our practice and consistent within the application of ethical frameworks. Values vary according to individual experiences; they can be standards or principles that determine behaviour and can define an individual's priorities. However, when personal values and ethics are not in conflict the combination of these two together can form the basis of effective decision-making.

ACTIVITY 3.1

Take time to reflect and list what your own personal values are.

Consider what you think the sources of these values that you hold are.

3.3 Why are values and ethics relevant to nursing and my role as a nursing associate?

As suggested, values and ethics provide a set of principles which inform and guide your everyday professional clinical practice and decision-making within healthcare, as well as guiding your personal behaviours. Similarly, our service users/patients also have their own values and beliefs and, like your own, these are based on their education, family background, peer influences and cultural and ethnicity characteristics. We need to respect these so that we provide safe, effective, non-discriminatory and compassionate person-centred care (NMC, 2018b).

The professional values for our everyday practice are set out in the NMC (2018a) *Code* and you must follow these professional values as a registered nursing associate, otherwise you may be subject to NMC fitness to practise proceedings. In addition, by the end of your programme of study, you must meet all the requirements of the NMC (2018b) *Standards* in order to become a registered nursing associate. Furthermore, in England, you need to abide by the 6Cs (DH, 2012) which are discussed in more detail later in this chapter.

In summary, values and ethics are core to your clinical practice so that you deliver care that is competent, compassionate, safe, respects each individual service user/patient and maintains their dignity.

ACTIVITY 3.2

What values do you think are important within the nursing profession?

Now compare these to your own personal values, as listed in *Activity 3.1*. Are there any values that conflict?

Consider how you might reconcile any potential conflicting values within your nursing practice.

3.4 Virtue ethics in everyday healthcare

Virtue theory was developed by Aristotle (384–322 BC), and Stohr (2006) states that this theory is taking precedence within medical and nursing ethics as the theory is concerned with an individual's character and integrity, which is the central focus of moral concern. Someone who shows virtues such as kindness, generosity, respect for persons, honesty and compassion will be the model of moral conduct (Campbell *et al.*, 1997). For virtue theorists the central question of morality is 'what kind of person ought I be?' and not 'what ought I to do?' Due to the person-centred nature, the virtues are the heart of our moral reasoning as it is the character of the person that can determine which action is to be taken. For example, an honest person is not just someone who performs honest acts; it is also their natural disposition that is an established habit.

Originally Aristotle outlined four cardinal virtues – courage, temperance, prudence and justice – which he considered to be of the utmost importance for morality. Aristotle viewed that over time the routine (habitual) practice of these virtues enabled an individual to act in a good way when faced with a moral dilemma. He explained this as 'phrenesis' or practical wisdom. The habitual practice of all these virtues would lead an individual to eudemonia (happiness or wellbeing) and to flourish as a human being. So, the question you may ask yourself is, how do you know when you are acting virtuously? Aristotle's 'doctrine of the mean' suggests that someone's character lies between two extremes. For example, if courage is the virtue, cowardice is a vice resulting from lack of courage, and recklessness is a vice resulting from an excess of courage. Therefore, to be courageous would be to act somewhere between these two extremes.

As societal norms have evolved and changed over time, what we deem virtuous has also changed and evolved. Although some universal virtues may remain, such as honesty, courage and justice, ethicists such as Rachels (1999) and Hursthouse (1999) identify benevolence, self-control, kindness and compassion as an evolution of these original virtues.

As a nursing associate it is important to acknowledge the ways in which virtues can support your practice. What lie at the core of moral behaviour are not rules and conduct but human qualities, such as the virtue of *caring*. For nursing associates, trustworthiness, quality of care and sensitivity in the face of service users'/patients' problems, needs and vulnerabilities are integral to the profession and the virtue of care (Beauchamp and Childress, 2019). An example is whether to break or maintain confidentiality and how you perform these actions; what motivation and feelings underlie this decision and how would the action promote or prevent positive patient relationships?

Earlier in the chapter we discussed the importance of professional values. Rassin (2008) suggests that values represent the basic convictions of what is right, good or desirable, and motivate both social and professional behaviour. Virtue ethics links closely with the 6Cs (care, compassion, courage, communication, competence and commitment), identified as 'fundamental values' in nursing care (DH, 2012).

>> **The 6Cs have been identified as fundamental values in nursing care.** These six values represent the professional behaviour expected within all healthcare practice, with courage as a core virtue.

An example of you being courageous as a nursing associate is in relation to safeguarding people who are vulnerable, raising concerns about standards of care or challenging accepted practices and implementing change. The NHS Constitution expects all NHS staff to raise concerns (NHS England, 2015) and it is a professional requirement for nurses to raise concerns about people who may be at risk. This is expressed within the NMC (2018a) *Code* and Platform 5 of the NMC (2018b, p. 10) *Standards* which identifies that you need to "identify risks to safety or experience and take appropriate action, putting the best interests, needs and preferences of people first".

In a different context you may also need to develop courage when supporting patients to face their own suffering and vulnerability. Without the courage to stay with a patient who is suffering, you may create distance from the patient which could lead to a lack of compassion; for example, end-of-life care. In all cases where the virtues can be applied the doctrine of the 'mean' needs to be remembered, in that the virtue needs to be between the two extremes. Thorup *et al.* (2012), like Aristotle, suggest that courage is developed over time (as with all virtues). Habitual practice and being caring, compassionate and courageous within your nursing practice will support you in working within the range of virtue ethics.

3.5 The four principles in everyday healthcare

Beauchamp and Childress (2019), who have been influential in healthcare ethics since the 1970s, proposed four principles of autonomy, beneficence, non-maleficence and justice. These are also referred to as 'principlism' and they form an ethical framework. This is not designed as a moral theory; rather the framework determines what one *ought to do*. Gillon (1994) states that the four-principle approach provides a simple, accessible and culturally neutral approach to thinking about ethical issues in healthcare by offering a common basic moral analytical framework with a common moral language. The principles are referred to as basic *prima facie* moral commitments. The *prima facie* principle, i.e. the one that is most valid, is one that is binding unless it conflicts with another principle – a situation that often occurs within nursing practice. Therefore, the goal using this ethical framework is to develop, specify and balance these principles against the moral dilemma in question.

3.5.1 Autonomy

Autonomy is the right that an individual has to make their own decisions and choices. Gillon (1986, p. 6) describes it as "the capacity to think, decide and act on the basis of such thought and decision... freely and independently without let or hindrance". Beauchamp and Childress (2019) define it as "self-rule that is free from both controlling interference of others and limitations that prevent meaningful choice, such as inadequate understanding. The autonomous individual acts freely in accordance with a self-chosen plan" (ibid, pp. 101–102). Alternative words for autonomy that we could use are independence, individuality and being one's own person (Cuthbert and Quallington, 2017).

As a nursing associate you are obliged to respect an individual's autonomy of thought, autonomy of will and autonomy of action. To be able to do this, we need to remember that individuals can think for themselves and have their own personal values, desires and aspirations. They are able to weigh up the advantages and disadvantages of a situation for themselves and decide what is the most appropriate action for them to take (Cuthbert and Quallington, 2017). At times, within healthcare, this means we may not agree with the patient's personal decision, but we still need to recognise it is their right to choose (NMC, 2018a); for example, if a patient decides to stop all their treatment for cancer which may lead to them dying sooner.

The principle of autonomy is embedded throughout the NMC (2018a) *Code*. The first section identifies that you need to 'prioritise people' within your scope of practice. Important points relating to autonomy are included within each of the five subsections:

1. **Treat people as individuals and uphold their dignity.** This involves you delivering nursing care which is person-centred and upholds their human rights (set out in the Human Rights Act 1998, discussed in *Section 3.5.4*), while treating them with dignity, respect, kindness and compassion. The NMC *Code* specifically states you need to "avoid making assumptions and

recognise diversity <u>and individual choice</u>" (NMC, 2018a, p. 6). An example of maintaining dignity is ensuring a patient is screened from other patients and covered appropriately when being physically examined.

2. **Listen to people and respond to their preferences and concerns**. To enable the delivery of effective care you must work in partnership with the service user/patient so they can contribute to their own health and wellbeing; this respects their autonomy. Your role is to empower them to be able to share in decisions about how they will be treated and cared for, while also recognising that individuals may differ in how much they want to be involved in this decision-making process. Naidoo and Wills (2016, p. 75) define empowerment as "the act of acquiring power and the ability to make decisions and take control of one's life". An important point to remember within a healthcare setting is that it is easy for us to disempower our service users/patients; for example, by the daily ward routine when waking them up or when the lights go off on the ward at night, or in the use of hospital gowns.

3. **Make sure that people's physical, social and psychological needs are assessed and responded to**. This section again refers to working in partnership with your service user/patient and "helping them to access relevant health and social care, information and support when they need it" (NMC, 2018a, p. 8). Accessing relevant information means they can seek to maintain their independence while enabling them to make an informed choice that is right for them. For example, you could provide information on weight loss verbally or with leaflets, or signpost them to information such as slimming clubs, dietitian, etc.

4. **Act in the best interests of people at all times**. As a nursing associate you are required to ensure that a service user/patient is fully informed and has agreed to any action. This is informed consent which needs to be documented. Any information that is given to them must be truthful and accurate and include possible consequences. It needs to be presented in a way they will understand; for instance, avoiding using 'health jargon' or ensuring the information is provided in their own language. One example is consent for an operation or treatment. As noted previously, you may need to respect a person's right to either agree to the treatment or to refuse it (NMC, 2018a, p. 7). There is also a need to balance your views about the decisions an individual chooses to make. You may not impose personal opinions, including moral, political and religious views on service users/patients. In addition, you are required to tell a service user/patient if you have a conscientious objection to a procedure they are to receive, as well as advising your manager and colleagues and arranging for another appropriately qualified nurse to provide the required care. There are very few and specific circumstances where it is possible to make a conscientious objection.

5. **Respect people's right to privacy and confidentiality**. As a nursing associate this means not only respecting your service user/patient's right to privacy (for example, drawing curtains around their bed) but also maintaining their confidentiality. They need to be informed about how their personal information will be used and shared with the people caring for them and their families (an exception is where patient safety or protection of the public is concerned; for example, safeguarding children or vulnerable adults). Sharing of data is also governed by national legislation within the Data Protection Act (2018) and locally by the Caldicott Principles (UK Caldicott Guardian Council, 2017).

ACTIVITY 3.3

Choose one of the NMC (2018a) *Code* clauses in the 'Prioritise people' section and note down some examples from clinical practice where you have seen autonomy being demonstrated.

3.5.2 Beneficence

Beauchamp and Childress (2019) state that the term beneficence denotes acts or qualities of mercy, kindness and compassion. These are actions of doing good and include all norms (something that is considered the standard), characters (motivations and intentions) and actions (behaviour) with the goal of benefiting or promoting the wellbeing of others.

The "principle of beneficence demands more than non-maleficence as agents need to take positive steps to help others, not merely refrain from harmful acts" (Beauchamp and Childress, 2019, p. 217). It is therefore the moral obligation to act in a way that benefits others. The principle of beneficence is integral to the nursing profession in order to alleviate pain and suffering, as well as to promote care and wellbeing. According to Beauchamp and Childress (2019) beneficence can be conceptualised as three principles; one ought to prevent harm or pain, one ought to remove harm or pain, and one ought to do or promote good. Beneficence supports an array of *prima facie* rules of obligation (Beauchamp and Childress, 2019).

Within the NMC (2018a) *Code*, the principle of beneficence is identified primarily within the first section of the need to 'prioritise people' within your scope of practice. As a nursing associate you are obliged to always act in the patient's best interest in your practice (Cuthbert and Quallington, 2017; NMC, 2018a), as we have discussed earlier. The principle of beneficence is the basis of the caring ethic of working in the best interests of patients as you are acting for the benefit of others. Beneficence can be demonstrated by helping others;

for example, helping an elderly person cross a road. Such acts need not be obligatory, but many people feel a moral obligation to help that is often triggered by an emotional response to act, that can be based on personal or professional moral values.

As a nursing associate you need to be able to *"balance* the need to act in the best interests of people at all times with the requirement to respect a person's right to accept or refuse treatment" (NMC, 2018a, p. 8). This includes acting as an advocate for the vulnerable as well as protecting and supporting service users/ patients who lose their autonomy, because of their physical or mental health or due to an injury, to choose. The legislation relating to this that you must follow is the Mental Capacity Act (DH, 2005) and the subsequent amendment made to this Act and the Liberty Protection Safeguards (LPS). However, there is difficulty in implementing the principle of beneficence, as the determining of what exactly is good for another and who can best make this decision can provide ethical dilemmas. Often these ethical dilemmas will require you to balance and consider what it is in *their* (service users'/patients') best interests and not what *we* (healthcare professionals) may *think* is in their best interests.

ACTIVITY 3.4

Reflect on your experience in clinical practice and consider a situation where there was an ethical dilemma between what the service users/patients wanted and what the healthcare professionals thought was in their best interests.

How was this situation resolved?

Paternalism

The ethical principles of beneficence and autonomy can conflict within nursing care, with the dilemma of whether respecting the autonomy of patients should have priority over beneficence; paternalistic beneficence remains a crucial problem within nursing care. Buchanan (1978) defines paternalism as an intentional interference with a person's preferences, desires or actions, such as the deliberate dissemination of misinformation or withholding information with the intention of either preventing or reducing harm to, or benefiting that person, therefore overriding autonomy. This would be considered as a paternalistic act. For example, there may be rare instances in practice where informing a patient of the full truth may not be appropriate; for example, where a patient has a cognitive impairment such as dementia and may not be competent to receive it. However, the NMC (2018b) *Standards* Platform 1.1.3 states the importance of courage, transparency and applying the Duty of Candour.

The Statutory Duty of Candour was introduced in 2014 and requires healthcare professionals to be open and honest with patients when things go wrong with their care or treatment. They must apologise when it does, and if possible, provide a remedy/solution, as well as explaining the short- and long-term effects of what has happened. All healthcare professionals have to be open and honest with their employers, colleagues, relevant organisations and regulators (for example, the NMC) and participate fully in any investigations or reviews. The Duty of Candour also means that you must raise any concerns when appropriate and support your colleagues to be open and honest as well (NMC and General Medical Council, 2015).

ACTIVITY 3.5

Read the NMC and General Medical Council (2015) *Openness and honesty when things go wrong: the professional duty of candour.* Available at: www.nmc.org.uk/globalassets/sitedocuments/nmc-publications/openness-and-honesty-professional-duty-of-candour.pdf or bit.ly/3ZgquQf

As nursing associates, it is important to understand paternalism and to know when paternalistic acts occur, as fundamentally the service user/patient is the only person who can decide what is good and what matters to themselves. Nursing associates can identify when a patient's autonomy has been diminished and should do everything possible to restore it. The outcome would then result in the principles of beneficence and autonomy being used in partnership rather than in conflict.

3.5.3 Non-maleficence

Non-maleficence is the obligation to abstain from causing harm to others; "above all or first do no harm" (Beauchamp and Childress, 2019, p. 155). This is the fundamental principle in the Hippocratic oath as it incorporates the obligation of non-maleficence and beneficence. The idea of benefiting others while not injuring or inflicting harm creates conflict between the two principles, as the principle of non-maleficence is the obligation to do no harm, which is distinct from the obligation to help or enable others. Often within healthcare as healthcare professionals you may inflict a minor injury such as swelling from a needle, but the benefit of saving a life is greater; in this instance the obligation of beneficence would take priority.

Non-maleficence at times can override other principles, but the weight of these principles will vary according to different ethical situations and dilemmas. However, it is important to note that no rule in ethics favours avoiding harm over providing benefit. Non-maleficence requires only "intentional avoidance of actions that cause harm" (Beauchamp and Childress, 2019, p. 157). Although the concept of non-maleficence has been explained, the understanding of what constitutes a harm is fundamental to professional practice. Beauchamp and Childress (2019) state that harm is a thwarting, defeating or a setting back of individuals' interests, but explain that a harmful action is not always wrong or unjustified.

Non-maleficence is a *prima facie* principle which cannot be viewed as an absolute (viewed without relation to other things; for example, good or evil are absolutes as you are either good or evil). This principle requires explicit justification if harmful actions occur, as long as the justification does not disregard the core moral obligation of non-maleficence; that is, not to kill. As a nursing associate you are obliged to *do no harm* and, as already stated, to always act in the patient's best interests in your practice (Cuthbert and Quallington, 2017). The principle of non-maleficence is identified in the NMC (2018a) *Code* in the section 'Preserve safety'. You need to address this principle within your scope of practice as it requires you to ensure that patient and public safety is not affected (also see NMC (2018b) *Standards* Platform 5).

Below, the core sections have been applied to the moral obligations of non-maleficence by Beauchamp and Childress (2019, p. 159):

- Do not kill

By recognising and working within the limits/scope of your competence you can ensure that no undue harm will be caused by accurately identifying, observing and assessing signs of a person receiving care, ensuring timely referrals as well as seeking the support of experienced professionals to carry out actions or procedures that go beyond your competence.

- Do not cause pain or suffering and do not incapacitate

Alongside ensuring you work within your limits and capabilities as a nursing associate, it is vital that you remain open and candid with all service users about all aspects of care and treatment, including when any mistakes or harm have taken place. This also supports the NMC (2018b) *Standards* Platform 1.1.3, which states the importance of being courageous and transparent, and applying the Duty of Candour.

Beauchamp and Childress (2019) discuss the issue of negligence and standard of due care. This is not only embedded within the law and NMC (2018a) *Code*, but is also a moral responsibility that due care and appropriate action are taken to avoid causing harm. Negligence is referred to as either intentionally or unintentionally imposing unreasonable or carelessly imposing risks of harm to a service user/patient. For example: a nurse knowingly failing to change a bandage as scheduled, creating an increased risk of infection is an intentional harm, whereas if the service user/patient tells you information that is personal and you forget that it's personal and discuss this with other nurses and it causes the service user/patient to be upset or embarrassed, this is an unintentional harm.

- Do not cause offence and do not deprive others of the goods of life

The NMC (2018a, p. 17) *Code* states the importance of raising concerns immediately if you believe a person is vulnerable or at risk of harm and needs extra support and protection. This also includes taking reasonable steps to protect and safeguard vulnerable individuals and those at risk of harm, and this may include knowing when to disclose information. If disclosure is deemed necessary this may diminish an individual's autonomy; however, it is on the premise of beneficence while adhering to the principle of non-maleficence by working in line with the legal parameters of disclosure which include removing a person from a risk of harm.

ACTIVITY 3.6

The NMC website states that "Being fit to practise requires a nurse, midwife or nursing associate to have the skills, knowledge, health and character to do their job safely and effectively". They will investigate the fitness to practise of registrants if allegations are made that they have not met the NMC standards for skills, education and behaviour.

Read their approach to fitness to practise, available at www.nmc.org.uk/concerns-nurses-midwives/fitness-to-practise-a-new-approach or bit.ly/3SDXq2E

3.5.4 Justice

Peate and Wild (2012, p. 98) explain that the ethical principle of justice is where "everyone is valued equally and treated alike". This means justice is about fairness, and Cuthbert and Quallington (2017) state that it is "a group of norms for distributing benefits and costs fairly" (ibid, p. 27). Distributive justice identifies that resources could be used in different ways, and Benbow *et al.* (2019, p. 74) suggest the following ways that these resources could be allocated in healthcare:

- "equal share to everyone
- random distribution
- on a first come, first served basis
- according to need
- to deserving cases
- to treat as many as possible".

ACTIVITY 3.7

Consider the above list. What would be the outcome for service users/patients in each of these six options?

Would they be fair to everyone?

In the UK the National Health Service (NHS) provides healthcare for all, so service users/patients receive free primary and secondary care when they need it. They do not have to pay for this care directly as it is funded by the government from taxation. The NHS Constitution (NHS England, 2015) sets out the principles and values for the NHS in England which includes fairness, as well as the expected behaviours of both service users/patients and staff:

> *"the rights to which patients, public and staff are entitled and pledges which the NHS is committed to achieve, together with responsibilities which the public, patients and staff owe to one another to ensure that the NHS operates fairly and effectively. The Secretary of State for Health, all NHS bodies, private and voluntary sector providers supplying NHS services, and local authorities in the exercise of their public health functions are required by law to take account of this Constitution in their decisions and actions." (NHS England, 2015).*

The principle of justice is also embedded within the NMC (2018a) *Code*. It states that, as nursing associates, you must "act with honesty and integrity at all times, treating people fairly and without discrimination, bullying or harassment" (ibid, 20.2, p. 21). You are also required to "keep to the laws of the country in which you are practising" (ibid, 20.4, p. 21) and there are many laws which relate to promoting fairness and discrimination.

In relation to this, as already noted, there is important legislation which you must follow: the Human Rights Act and the Equality Act.

Human Rights Act

The Human Rights Act (1998) sets out in law what every individual has a right to expect regarding their personal human rights and freedoms. This is regardless of their age, gender, disability, ethnic identity, sexuality or social class. These are called protected characteristics as they are protected by law. It is against the law for public authorities (the NHS and local authorities), you as a nursing associate, and all health and social care workers, to act in a way which is contrary to the fourteen articles contained within the Act. Those most relevant to you when delivering nursing care are:

- Article 8: Right to respect for private and family life, home and correspondence

- Article 9: Freedom of thought, conscience and religion
- Article 14: Freedom from discrimination.

Equality Act

The Human Rights Act provided the basis for the Equality Act (2010). This Act is the law which protects and promotes equal opportunities for all and makes it illegal to discriminate. This may be in the form of direct discrimination or indirect discrimination. Direct discrimination means treating a person deliberately differently from someone else because of their gender, disability, ethnic identity, sexuality or social class. Indirect discrimination may be as a result of organisational policies or practice policy which are applied to everyone but, in reality, disadvantages a group of people who share one or more of the protected characteristics specified above. This would apply whether in a hospital, other workplace or within the wider population.

The NMC (2018b) *Standards* specify that by the end of the programme you will be able to:

> *"1.11 provide, promote, and where appropriate advocate for, non-discriminatory, person-centred and sensitive care at all times. Reflect on people's values and beliefs, diverse backgrounds, cultural characteristics, language requirements, needs and preferences, taking account of any need for adjustments" (ibid, p. 5).*

Furthermore, the NMC (2018a, p. 21: 20.2) *Code* states that you must "act with honesty and integrity at all times, treating people fairly and without discrimination, bullying or harassment". Therefore, you must uphold justice/fairness and the law every day in your clinical practice, both as a trainee nursing associate and when you are a registered nursing associate.

RECAP

- Values and ethics are relevant to healthcare as they provide a set of principles which inform and guide your everyday professional clinical practice.
- The four principles proposed by Beauchamp and Childress are:
  - Autonomy: the right that an individual has to make their own decisions and choices
  - Beneficence: the moral obligation to act in a way that benefits others
  - Non-maleficence: the obligation to do no harm to others
  - Justice: the ethical principle of valuing everyone equally and treating everyone alike.
- These principles often conflict with one another and they must be balanced against the moral dilemma in question.

3.6 Accountability

Accountability can be defined as "being liable for what you have, or have not done, and to give an account of your decisions" (Benbow *et al.*, 2019, p. 31). This means you can be asked in your role as a nursing associate to explain your actions or non-actions and are responsible for those decisions. Being accountable for your practice is a way in which the public are protected.

Platform 1 of the NMC (2018b) *Standards* is entitled "Being an accountable professional". Within this platform, the outcomes explain the proficiencies you need to develop and apply to all the standards of proficiencies in platforms 2–6. These all need to be achieved at the point of your registration with the NMC after successfully completing your programme of study (NMC, 2018b, pp. 4–6). As previously discussed, the NMC (2018b, p. 4) *Standards* state that nursing associates must "act in the best interest of people, putting them first and providing care that is person-centred, safe and compassionate". In addition, nursing associates must "act professionally at all times and use their knowledge and experience to make evidence based decisions and solve problems. They recognise and work within the limits of their competence and are responsible for their actions" (ibid., p. 4).

ACTIVITY 3.8

Read all the outcomes set out within Platform 1 of the NMC (2018b) *Standards of Proficiency for Nursing Associates*.

List who you are responsible for and accountable to in your role as a nursing associate.

Outcome 1.1. clearly states that you must "understand and act in accordance with the [NMC] *Code*" (NMC, 2018b, p. 5). When you successfully complete your programme, you must register with the NMC in order to practise as a nursing associate. As part of this you make a declaration of good health and good character and are required to maintain your registration by completing the revalidation process every three years (for more information and ensuring you remain in good health and character, see www.nmc.org.uk/revalidation).

You have a duty of care to your service users/patients and their carers to deliver care to an 'appropriate standard'. Cuthbert and Quallington's (2017) explanation is clearer when you look at this from a negative perspective. You can be held responsible if you fail to give care that meets the required standards and this failure means the service user/patient suffers "distress, harm, humiliation, fear, neglect or simply loss of trust" (non-maleficence) (ibid., p. 215).

You will see that 1.2 (NMC, 2018b, p. 5) requires you to "understand and apply relevant legal, regulatory and governance requirements, policies, and ethical frameworks, including any mandatory reporting duties, to all areas of practice". Therefore, you must apply the ethical principles to your clinical practice, as outlined in this chapter, together with following your employing organisation's policies and procedures and abiding by the laws of the country in which you practise. In addition, you are accountable to your employer and you will have a contract of employment which sets out your rights and responsibilities within the organisation and their expectations of you which you must follow. This also includes your obligation to undertake all mandatory (core skills) training which you are required to do both as a trainee nursing associate and as a registered nursing associate.

Furthermore, you are accountable under both criminal and civil law. Under criminal law you are accountable for any action that the law of the country forbids. This would need to be proved in the criminal courts; for example, murder or manslaughter, racial harassment (Benbow *et al.*, 2019). Civil law covers the rights and duties that all individuals have to each other; for example, injunctions which stop a person acting unlawfully against another or compensation for damages (Benbow *et al.*, 2019). Hence, the NMC requires you to have an indemnity arrangement which covers your scope of practice.

> » **Your contract of employment sets out your rights and responsibilities within the organisation and your employer's expectations of you.**

As a nursing associate you are also accountable to your colleagues, not only to communicate effectively with them both verbally and through accurate and timely record-keeping (which is a legal requirement), but also to actively collaborate with them in multidisciplinary teams and with the service user/patient, to deliver quality care which is safe and in the service user's/patient's best interests. Platform 4 of the NMC (2018b, pp. 12–13) *Standards* identifies the proficiencies you need to be able to work effectively as a member of the team. Platform 6 (NMC, 2018b, pp. 16–17) sets out the proficiencies required for you to contribute to integrated care and caring for people with complex needs, working with different agencies and interdisciplinary teams.

As a reminder, in your role as a trainee nursing associate and registered nursing associate you are required to raise any concerns that you have (see Duty of Candour which is discussed in *Section 3.5.2*) relating to "recognising and reporting any situations, behaviours or errors that could result in poor care outcomes" (NMC, 2018b, p. 5). As a trainee nursing associate you will be given the protocol for how to raise concerns from your training organisation and, as a registered nursing associate, your employing organisation will have its own policy and protocol. You are also expected to report any discriminatory behaviour that you observe (NMC, 2018b, p.5).

ACTIVITY 3.9

Watch the following *NMC Caring with Confidence: the code in action* bite-size animations, available at: www.nmc.org.uk/standards/code/code-in-action

Please ensure you read all the NMC (2018a) *Code* in full, as only selected clauses are discussed in this chapter. Finally, remember that throughout your career as a nursing associate you must abide by the standards set out in this Code.

CHAPTER SUMMARY

- Understanding your own personal values, and how you are motivated and driven by your own core values, is important within your personal life and your professional nursing practice.
- The knowledge and understanding of your own personal values will support you in your role as nursing associate in distinguishing between personal and professional values.
- The fundamental professional nursing values are human dignity, equality among patients and prevention of suffering, as well as integrity, altruism and honesty.
- You must provide safe, effective, non-discriminatory and compassionate person-centred care adhering to the Nursing and Midwifery Council (NMC) (2018a) *The Code: professional standards of practice and behaviour for nurses, midwives and nursing associates* and the 6Cs (DH, 2012).

FURTHER READING

Cuthbert, S. and Quallington, J. (2017) *Values and Ethics for Care Practice*. Lantern Publishing.

Duncan, P. (2010) *Values, Ethics and Health Care*. SAGE.

Seedhouse, D. (2009) *Ethics: the heart of healthcare*, 3rd edition. Wiley-Blackwell.

References

Beauchamp, T. and Childress, J. (2019) *Principles of Biomedical Ethics*, 8th edition. Oxford University Press.

Benbow, W., Jordan, G., Knight, A. and White, S. (2019) *A Handbook for Student Nurses: introducing key issues relevant for practice*, 3rd edition. Lantern Publishing.

Buchanan, A. (1978) Medical paternalism. *Philosophy and Public Affairs*, 7(4): 370–90.

Campbell, A.V., Charlesworth, M., Gillet, G. and Jones, G. (1997) *Medical Ethics*. Oxford University Press.

Cuthbert, S. and Quallington, J. (2017) *Values and Ethics for Care Practice*. Lantern Publishing.

Data Protection Act (2018) Available at: www. legislation.gov.uk/ukpga/2018/12/contents/ enacted (accessed 4 December 2022).

DH (2005) Mental Capacity Act. Available at: www.legislation.gov.uk/ukpga/2005/9/contents (accessed 4 December 2022).

DH (2012) *Compassion in Practice: nursing, midwifery and care staff – our vision and strategy.* Available at: www.england.nhs.uk/wp-content/uploads/2012/12/compassion-in-practice.pdf or bit.ly/3J45x5o (accessed 4 December 2022)

Duncan, P. (2010) *Values, Ethics and Health Care.* SAGE.

Dworkin, R. (1995) *Life's Dominion: an argument about abortion, euthanasia, and individual freedom.* Harper Collins.

Equality Act (2010) Available at: www.legislation.gov.uk/ukpga/2010/15/2020-03-19 (accessed 4 December 2022).

Gillon, R. (1986) *Philosophical Medical Ethics.* Wiley.

Gillon, R. (1994) Medical ethics: four principles plus attention to scope. *British Medical Journal,* **309** (6948): 184–8.

Halstead, J.M. and Reiss, M.J. (2003) *Values in Sex Education: from principles to practice.* RoutledgeFalmer.

Human Rights Act (1998) Available at: www.legislation.gov.uk/ukpga/1998/42/contents (accessed 4 December 2022).

Hursthouse, R. (1999) *On Virtue Ethics.* Open University Press.

Mehmet, N. (2011) 'Ethics and Wellbeing'. In A. Knight and A. McNaught (eds) (2011) *Understanding Wellbeing: an introduction for students and practitioners of health and social care.* Lantern Publishing.

Naidoo, J. and Wills, J. (2016) *Foundations for Health Promotion,* 4th edition. Elsevier.

NHS England (2015) *NHS Constitution for England.* Available at: www.gov.uk/government/publications/the-nhs-constitution-for-england or bit.ly/3J0qIp0 (accessed 4 December 2022).

NMC (2018a) *The Code: professional standards of practice and behaviour for nurses, midwives and nursing associates.* Nursing and Midwifery Council.

NMC (2018b) *Standards of Proficiency for Nursing Associates.* Nursing and Midwifery Council.

NMC and General Medical Council (2015) *Openness and honesty when things go wrong: the professional duty of candour.* Available at: www.nmc.org.uk/globalassets/sitedocuments/nmc-publications/openness-and-honesty-professional-duty-of-candour.pdf or bit.ly/3Y9KtPg (accessed 4 December 2022).

Oxford English Dictionary, 3rd edition (2010) Oxford University Press.

Peate, I. and Wild, K. (eds) (2012) *Nursing Practice: knowledge and care.* Wiley-Blackwell.

Poorchangizi, B., Borhani, F., Abbaszadeh, A. Mirzaee, M. and Farokhzadian, J. (2019) The importance of professional values from nursing students' perspective. *BMC Nursing,* **18**(26): 1–7.

Rachels, J. (1999) *The Elements of Moral Philosophy.* McGraw-Hill International.

Rassin, M. (2008) Nurses' professional and personal values. *Nursing Ethics,* **15**(5): 614–30.

Stohr, K. (2006) Contemporary virtue ethics. *Philosophy Compass,* **1**(1): 22–7.

Thorup, C. B., Rundqvist, E., Roberts, C. and Delmar, C. (2012) Care as a matter of courage: vulnerability, suffering and ethical formation in nursing care. *Scandinavian Journal of Caring Science,* **26**(3): 427–35.

UK Caldicott Guardian Council (2017) *A Manual for Caldicott Guardians.* Available at: www.ukcgc.uk/manual/contents (accessed 4 December 2022).

SOCIETY AND ITS IMPACT ON HEALTH

David Matthews

This chapter relates to outcomes 1.11, 2.4, 2.5, 2.6, 3.1 and 3.2 within the *Standards of Proficiency for Nursing Associates* (NMC, 2018).

LEARNING OUTCOMES

When you have completed this chapter you should be able to:
- Understand that the concept of health is not fixed, but that there exist competing models.
- Recognise that the experience of health and wellbeing is not just a biological issue, but is greatly determined by society.
- Have an awareness of key social determinants of health and wellbeing.
- Understand how good and bad health, alongside wellbeing more generally, is unequally distributed among social groups as a result of their social circumstances.

4.1 Introduction

The purpose of this chapter is to provide an overview of how society influences the health of individuals. It will be demonstrated that health is unequally distributed throughout society as a result of varying social circumstances people experience. Biology dominates our knowledge of health. Differences in health between individuals are frequently assumed to initially be a result of biological variation. However, as significant as biology is, social experiences are also greatly influential. As Marmot (2016) argues, health cannot be left to doctors alone. Rather it must be accepted that the social conditions within which individuals are born, develop as children, work and age, have significant consequences for health (Marmot, 2016). There is indeed little evidence to suggest that poor health is caused purely by biological phenomena operating in isolation from social factors (White, 2017).

4.2 Social determinants of health

When discussing how society contributes to the experience of health, and how social factors shape and organise both good and poor health, reference is frequently made to the social determinants of health. These are those social, political and economic factors that influence the health of individuals, communities and populations (Humber, 2019). Accepting them as significant, the World Health Organization (WHO) defined the social determinants of health as "the conditions in which people are born, grow, work, live and age, and people's access to power, money and resources. The social determinants are the major drivers of health inequities" (WHO, 2021a). For the WHO, the social determinants of health greatly determine the opportunity for all individuals to achieve good physical and mental health. In response to Covid-19, the distribution of which, the WHO argued, was greatly influenced by the social determinants of health, the WHO argued that individuals with enhanced living and working conditions, higher levels of education, and good access to health and welfare services, had a better opportunity of protecting themselves from Covid-19 (WHO, 2021a).

ACTIVITY 4.1

Why do you think enhanced access to, and a good experience of, the following factors might have provided added protection from Covid-19?
- Living conditions
- Working environment
- Education
- Health and welfare services

For Dahlgren and Whitehead (1991), there exist varying social determinants of health, ranging from those considered to be related more to lifestyle and behavioural issues (more about which can be found in the chapter on public health and health promotion), to others which are largely the result of the way society operates and is organised (*Figure 4.1*). Given their breadth, it is not possible in a single chapter to cover them all. Consequently, three of the most significant social determinants will be examined here, these being determinants which all nursing associates are likely to experience, in varying ways, as impacting upon the health of their service users. These determinants are:

1. Social class
2. Gender
3. Ethnicity.

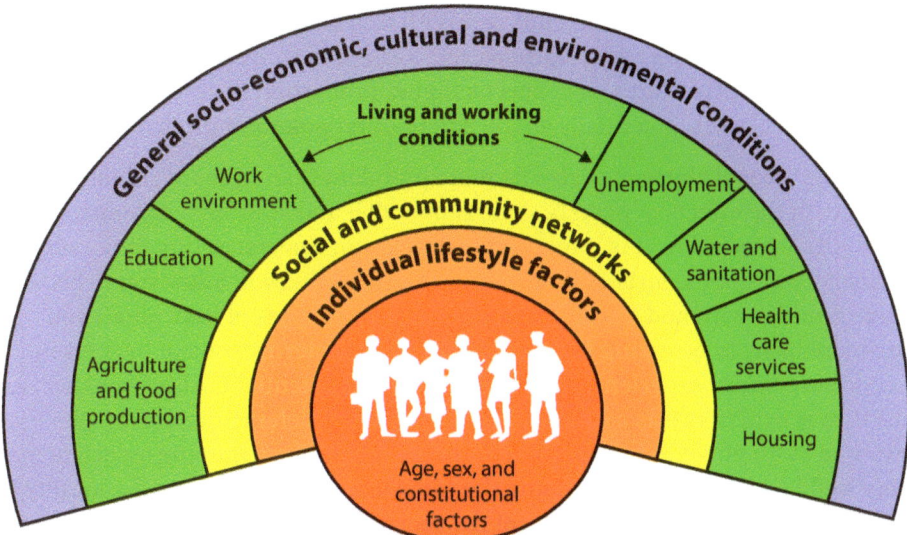

Figure 4.1: *The Dahlgren–Whitehead rainbow. Reproduced with permission from Institute for Futures Studies.*

Before examining how society influences the distribution of health, however, an argument will be made exemplifying why, as nursing associates, it is important for you to have an understanding of how society influences health.

4.3 Why society? Understanding your service users

Few would argue against the claim that fundamental to the provision of good quality care is ensuring that all service users are understood as individuals, having specific personality characteristics and needs which must be met. As such, an understanding of service users is essential if, as a nursing associate, you are to deliver the best service. An awareness of how society works is essential for this. Significant aspects of an individual's personality, identity and character, including their health, are influenced by social factors and the individual's place in society. Awareness of how social factors subsequently influence the distribution of health within the population is crucial for nursing associates, in order to understand how particular health issues are distributed among social groups, and broadly associated with individuals from different social backgrounds. The benefits of this awareness are particularly evident for nursing associates when considering the locality in which you work.

>> **Understanding your service users and how social factors influence their health is essential to deliver the best service.**

All localities have social characteristics. For example, it is commonly identified that some areas are affluent and some seen as deprived, while others can be considered as populated by members of different ethnic groups and characterised by different cultures. With this being so, all localities are dominated by particular social groups and social issues. By way of illustration, a hospital in a deprived area can expect a higher proportion of service users from lower social classes, potentially single parents, and possibly ethnic minorities.

Drug and alcohol abuse may also be more prevalent than in more affluent areas, along with the effects of poverty such as poor diet and substandard housing. As a nursing associate it is important to develop an understanding of the social characteristics of the locality in which you work, as this will allow you to become more familiar with and develop an awareness of the types of individuals you are more likely to be caring for, the specific social determinants of health your service users may experience, and the subsequent potential health issues service users may experience as a consequence of the social determinants they are exposed to. In effect, it is important to realise that being a nursing associate may very well be different, despite doing the same job, depending upon the locality where you work, as a consequence of the social characteristics of the locality and the impact of those characteristics on service users.

ACTIVITY 4.2

Think about the locality in which you are training. What are some of its social characteristics? Think about such things as wealth and poverty, the ethnic backgrounds of the people living there, their age profile, and so on.

RECAP

- The social determinants of health are those social, political and economic factors that influence the health of individuals, communities and populations.
- It is important to develop an understanding of your service users as individuals.
- An awareness of the social characteristics of the locality in which you work and the impact of those characteristics on service users is also important in delivering the best service to your users.

4.4 Biomedical model

While it might be thought that health is straightforward to understand, especially if it is considered a biological phenomenon, there is in fact no fixed understanding of it. Instead there are competing definitions and models of health which professionals draw upon to frame their perspectives and actions.

Two of the most dominant definitions of health are that of the biomedical model and social model, with the latter being the model adopted in this chapter.

The biomedical model, Barry and Yuill (2016) argue, is the primary way of understanding health. At the centre of this model is the human body and its biological composition, with poor health having its aetiological cause in the biological dysfunction of the body. All diseases, this model contends, have a biological cause which impacts upon the body in a universal and predictable manner. As a consequence, Germov (2012) asserts that, theoretically at least, there exist universal remedies, with the same 'cure' applied to everyone who experiences the same disease. With the cause of poor health being considered biological, it is subsequently the body which is the focus of attention in efforts to alleviate symptoms and correct problems. Medical professionals intervene, often with the use of medicines, drugs and operative procedures, directing their attention towards those aspects of the body which are thought to need correction. As a consequence, the biomedical model embraces and promotes the use of medical technology to treat poor health and encourage good health.

The biomedical model is commonly considered reductionist, reducing the cause of poor health to one single determinant, that of biology (White, 2017). As medical science has advanced, there has been an ever greater focus on increasingly smaller aspects of the human body, such as cells, molecules and genes as the causes of poor health, focusing more and more on these biological aspects at the expense of psychological and social causes.

ACTIVITY 4.3

Why do you think the biomedical model is the dominant way of understanding health in society?

4.5 Social model

In contrast to the biomedical model is the social model of health. Within the social science disciplines of sociology and social policy, as well as for many individuals in the fields of public health, health promotion and epidemiology, this model provides an alternative framework for understanding health, with the origins of poor health seen as something greatly influenced by society.

Over the last few decades, the causes of morbidity and mortality, globally, have increasingly been identified as the result of individuals acquiring chronic illnesses (Barry and Yuill, 2016). As of 2021, according to WHO, such diseases accounted for 71% of all global deaths, with cardiovascular disease, cancer, diabetes and respiratory issues amounting to 80% of all premature deaths caused by chronic illnesses (see *Table 4.1*). Such illnesses, however, do not largely originate from biological processes located within the body, but are the result of social conditions, circumstances and behaviour (White, 2017). They are therefore social in origin. Subsequently, we can talk of social pathology.

Table 4.1 *The main causes of death as a result of non-communicable disease in 2021 globally (WHO, 2021b)*

Non-communicable disease	Number of deaths
Cardiovascular disease	17.9 million
Cancers	9.3 million
Respiratory disease	4.1 million
Diabetes	1.5 million

Although not ignoring biology, the social model of health does not start with biological phenomena as the cause of poor health. It places health within a social context. The social model understands health to be influenced by social factors. They include, among other social causes, social class, working conditions, housing, the urban landscape, gender, ethnicity, and access to public services (see *Figure 4.2*). The social model contends that health is the result of the interaction between the individual and their social environment. With individuals experiencing various social conditions which are either conducive or detrimental to their health, it is the case that both good and poor health are unevenly distributed throughout society, with society being characterised by health inequalities where some groups in society are exposed to more negative social factors than other groups.

>> **The social model of health places health within a social context.**

From the perspective of the social model, methods to promote good health cannot rely upon biomedical interventions alone. Instead, they must focus upon the social circumstances of individuals, as well as wider social factors which are beyond the immediate influence of the individual, such as the availability of, and access to, public services and welfare support, reducing income inequality, provision of affordable housing, and greater access to educational opportunities, among many others.

ACTIVITY 4.4

Which health services in the UK do you think are influenced by the biomedical model of health and which services are influenced by the social model of health?

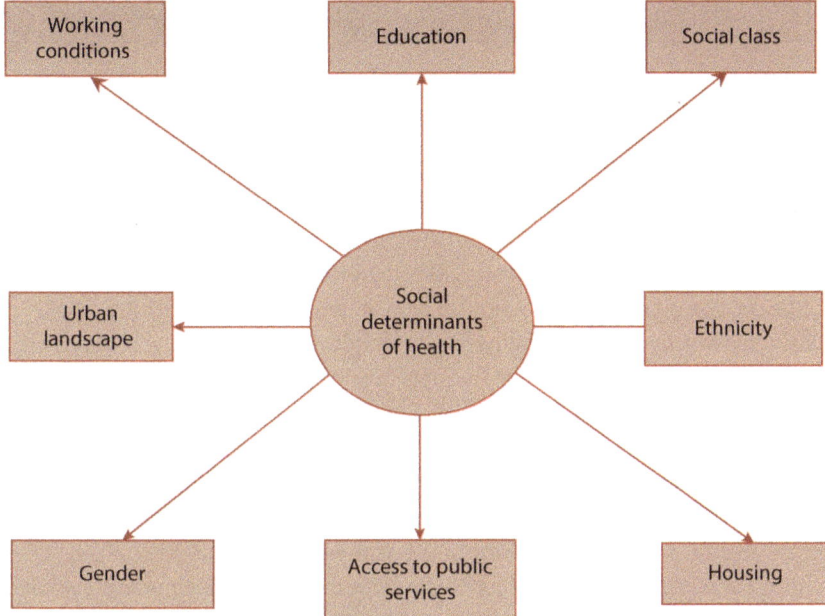

Figure 4.2 *Key social determinants of health.*

Accepting that social determinants play a role in influencing health is to accept the importance of the social model of health. Having discussed what is meant by the social determinants of health and the social model, we now need to examine in more detail how social class, gender and ethnicity can impact upon the health of individuals.

4.6 Social class, money and wealth

Various and often contested measurements of and efforts to define an individual's social class exist. Arguably one of the more common is that based upon the indicators of occupation and income. How income impacts upon health

» **Low income and poor working conditions have a detrimental impact on an individual's health.**

is significant, with a strong established relationship between low income and poor health (Marmot *et al.*, 2020). Further, there exists a definitive correlation between health and occupation, with insecure poorly paid employment and poor working conditions having a detrimental impact upon health and wellbeing, both physically and mentally (Marmot *et al.*, 2020). Overall, on average, in a country such as the UK, the less income an individual has, the poorer their health will be. This is known as the social gradient of health.

ACTIVITY 4.5

In what ways can insecure, poorly paid employment impact negatively upon someone's physical and mental health?

In the UK, a country which has high levels of income inequality, health inequalities can be dramatic. Between 2017 and 2019, in England, life expectancy (LE) for males living in the 10% most deprived neighbourhoods was an average of 74.1 years, compared to 83.5 years for males living in the wealthiest 10%. Similarly, for women in the most deprived neighbourhoods, LE was 78.7 years in comparison to 86.4 years for those living in the wealthiest neighbourhoods (ONS, 2021). Additionally, there exist significant variations in healthy life expectancy (HLE), which is the number of years an individual can expect to live in good health. In the most deprived localities in England, between 2017 and 2019, male and female HLE was 52.3 years and 51.4 years respectively, compared to 70.7 for males and 71.2 for females in the most affluent localities (ONS, 2021). The wealthiest men and women in the UK can expect to experience nearly two decades more of healthy life compared to the poorest. Statistically there exists a strong correlation between wealth and health, yet statistics tell us very little about the social circumstances which contribute to this pattern.

4.6.1 Materialism and the conditions of life

The manner in which social class and income influence the distribution of health can be illustrated with what are referred to as materialist factors. A materialist understanding of health focuses on those factors which influence the conditions in which individuals live and work (White, 2017). While materialist influences are plenty, of particular significance are occupation and working conditions, the physical organisation of the urban landscape, availability of and access to public services, educational opportunities, housing, exposure to pollution and environmental decline, and diet. More often, the unequal distribution of income influences the relationship between individuals and all these factors, with those on low incomes tending to be exposed to unhealthier material conditions.

Our modern understanding of a materialist approach to health originates from the investigations of Friedrich Engels (1845). Investigating the health conditions of the working class in England during the mid-nineteenth century, he argued that ill health was significantly influenced by the pursuit of profit; the majority of working class individuals in this time worked in dangerous circumstances, resulting in disability and sometimes death, and lived in overcrowded conditions spreading disease because of poverty.

Occupation can greatly impact an individual's health. Where people work in manual occupations, such as in heavy industry, in factories, or in construction, risks of injury and accidents are inevitably greater, despite the existence and growth of health and safety regulations over the last century in countries such as the UK. However, while many incidents of occupational mortality and morbidity are often associated with manual occupations positioned at the lower end of the social class spectrum, occupations thought to be middle class can also have negative consequences for an individual's health. White-collar occupations expose workers to increased risk of problems such as repetitive strain injury and the potential consequences of sedentary working conditions. Moreover, aside from the physical aspects, many individuals in a variety of jobs, be they manual or white-collar, may also feel a lack of control or autonomy at work, resulting in a sense of alienation which impacts upon their mental wellbeing (Matthews, 2019). On the other hand, more senior white-collar roles may potentially inflict great levels of stress on individuals, which, while having negative consequences for mental wellbeing, can also impact upon physical health such as increasing the risk of cardiovascular disease.

ACTIVITY 4.6

Which occupations and professions do you think have potentially negative consequences for an individual's health?

Alongside occupation, housing, which is one of the most important materialist factors for anyone, can have severe consequences for health. This is overwhelmingly determined by an individual's level of income. Poorer housing increases the risk of experiencing accidents as a result of overcrowding and unsafe conditions, while individuals have a greater chance of developing respiratory problems as a consequence of damp and poor air quality (White, 2017).

Related to housing, the impact of the wider built environment can have significant consequences for ill health. A locality's affluence impacts upon physical features, local resources and the socio-cultural environment (Annandale, 2014). The affluence or poverty of the urban environment influences the development of, and is illustrated by, the availability of public services, housing conditions, levels of pollution, rates of crime, and the quality of private sector enterprises in terms of the goods and services provided, such as takeaways, tanning salons and pawnbroking outlets, as well as access to green space such as parks. The affluence and poverty of space and place can have serious consequences for health.

ACTIVITY 4.7

If an individual lived in an area of a city where there existed high crime rates and increased levels of pollution, how might this impact upon their physical and mental health?

The impact of the urban landscape upon health has been illustrated by the Royal Society for Public Health (RSPH) (2018) in its identification of what constitutes a healthy town. To promote good health, healthy towns require high streets free from excess noise and pollution, architecturally designed to support activities such as walking and cycling, to be planned and provide services to facilitate social interaction and improve social cohesion and to encourage the establishment of businesses providing healthier services and goods. Crucially, the research identified a link between healthy high streets and local deprivation, with the localities of the ten unhealthiest exhibiting greater levels of deprivation than the ten healthiest (RSPH, 2018).

ACTIVITY 4.8

How important is social interaction for an individual's health?

4.7 Gender: men, women and health

It is observed that women have lower mortality rates than men (Annandale, 2014), but suffer greater morbidity (White, 2017). Moreover, certain health and wellbeing issues are commonly claimed to be associated with one gender more than another, with women experiencing greater levels of dementia, depression and arthritis, while men are more prone to lung cancer, cardiovascular disease and suicide (Broom, 2012).

>> **Biological differences may influence the different health status of men and women but they do not determine health differences.**

Attempts to explain gender variations commonly draw upon biological differences, with efforts to account for the health status of men and women illustrating supposed inherent biological differences. Consequently, biomedical interpretations often dominate efforts to explain gender health inequalities. This has given rise to the growth of gender-specific medicine utilising scientific analysis to explain variations in the physiological differences between the genders. Scientific analyses, however, can be criticised for overemphasising differences associated with gender. Biologically the division between men and women is far less than is popularly understood. It would, however, be unwise to dismiss the *influence* of biology on the health of men and women, but biology does not *determine* health differences (Annandale, 2014).

4.7.1 Women as caregivers

The extent to which society determines gender health inequalities is considerable. One influential argument is with regard to gender-specific roles men and women have within society. In relation to women, their role as a carer is identified as having great consequences for their health. Despite increasing involvement by men over the last three to four decades, it is the case that women remain the primary caregivers in society, having the responsibility for the majority of informal care of family members including children, disabled adults and the elderly. As Public Health England (now the UK Health Security Agency since October 2021) argued, a typical carer is likely to be female and in her 50s and 60s. The impact of this often difficult, challenging and time-consuming role on women can include reduced sleep, less leisure time, and increased risk of poverty, should a woman be a full-time carer. All three can have significant direct and indirect consequences for a woman's physical and mental health. Focusing on those who provide care for elderly individuals, Public Health England identified that the consequences of being a carer can include stress, anxiety and depression. Moreover, carers of all individuals who require care are at greater risk of cardiovascular disease, musculoskeletal conditions and cognitive decline (Public Health England, 2021).

Although an assertion which is contestable, women's status as dominant care providers has often been justified as a result of their reproductive function, which in itself has been medicalised. The days immediately prior to menstruation, for instance, are no longer viewed as a time of hormonal imbalance in the form of premenstrual tension (PMT), but a medical syndrome in the form of premenstrual syndrome (PMS) (Morrall, 2009). Over time, women's bodies have increasingly been exposed to the clinical gaze. Over the last half century, or more, women's bodies have been constructed as a medical issue more so than men's, meaning they are scrutinised and regulated more by medical professionals. An increasing medicalisation of women's bodies has meant women consult doctors more regularly and attend hospital more frequently than men (White, 2017).

ACTIVITY 4.9

Think: is more attention given by the medical profession to women's bodies than those of men?

Along with women's role as the main providers of care, medicalisation is a significant reason for women coming into contact more often with medical professionals and using the health system more than men. Outside childbearing age women have a tendency to attend hospital at the same rate as men (Broom, 2012), and when men and women are exposed to the same stressful non-gender-specific situations they have broadly the same rates of depression (Nazroo *et al.*, 1997). Therefore when these variables are no longer a factor or are controlled, gendered health inequalities are reduced.

4.7.2 Masculinity and femininity

How men and women are expected to behave is greatly determined by society's expectations, with this being influenced by the concepts of femininity and masculinity. Both of these concepts are social constructs, as what it means to be a man or woman is culturally and historically specific, and both concepts have consequences for health. The emphasis society places upon women, more than men, as the main providers of care is a construction of femininity by society. Further, societal pressures regarding femininity in terms of appearance can be identified as contributing to the greater prevalence of eating disorders amongst young women.

Constructions of masculinity can have just as negative consequences for men. In an effort to 'prove' themselves, young males have a tendency to be less risk-averse, taking part in such activities as contact sports, excessive alcohol consumption and dangerous driving. As a result males exhibit higher rates of both accidental and non-accidental injuries (Broom, 2012). Further, while it is claimed that women exhibit greater levels of mental health issues, men have a tendency to internalise anger, turning to substance and alcohol abuse as a source of relief, while women are more likely to express their feelings and seek support. For some men, especially teenage boys and young men, such pressures can be too much during the transition from adolescence to adulthood, potentially resulting in drug abuse or even suicide (White, 2017).

4.8 Ethnicity and health inequalities

The impact of social class upon the distribution of health has been recognised widely for well over a century, even if there have been at times, among some, a reluctance to acknowledge it. The relationship between gender and health has also long been accepted. However, conceding that ethnicity is also a determinant is a relatively recent phenomenon. Only since the 1970s has there been any serious attempt to both recognise and analyse its impact upon the social distribution of health (Karlsen and Nazroo, 2000).

Efforts to understand the extent to which ethnicity contributes to health are at times hampered and made more complex by the fact that ethnicity can prove difficult to determine. Broadly, ethnicity refers to the identification of population groups based upon social, cultural and historical variations. Ethnic groups are characterised by organised cultural boundaries such as language, religion and country of origin, which differentiate groups. Ethnicity is a subjective concept, consisting both of self-identification and categorisation by others. Individuals can recognise themselves as belonging to a particular group, with the way they subsequently act and think influencing the perception they have of their ethnicity. Thus ethnicity can be considered as an active construction of its members. At the same time individuals can be categorised as belonging to an ethnic group by others; they are therefore labelled as belonging to an ethnicity based upon others' interpretations. Ethnicity is consequently an arbitrary concept, with this presenting a challenge to health researchers.

ACTIVITY 4.10

What ethnicity do you consider yourself to be, and what are you drawing upon to differentiate yourself from people who you think are from different ethnic backgrounds from yourself?

4.8.1 Ethnicity as a health inequality

Historically, discussions relating to how ethnicity impacts upon health often focused on the role of biology and genetics, with it broadly argued that health differences between ethnic groups could be largely accounted for by biological and genetic variation among different ethnic groups (Barry and Yuill, 2016). Contemporary debates, however, dismiss this position. While the reasons for health variations between ethnic groups are contested, many professionals and academic disciplines reject emphatically biological and genetic interpretations due to the lack of evidence. Various global population groups may be characterised as possessing certain genes, but these predominantly influence hair, eye and skin colour and are of little importance with regard to the body's susceptibility to disease (Bartley, 2016). Global populations have far more biological and genetic commonalities than differences, and any variations which do exist are no greater than those that exist within one population group (White, 2017). Attempts to focus upon, and identify, biological and genetic causes for the ill health experienced by ethnic groups conjure up the real danger of falling into racist assertions.

>> **There is a lack of evidence to support the assertion that biological and genetic variation among different ethnic groups accounts for health disparities, and many professionals and academic disciplines reject this argument.**

Not uncommonly, as Barry and Yuill (2016) argue, certain health concerns have been associated with particular ethnic groups, with such claims often predicated upon assumptions of biological and genetic dispositions towards various health problems. Sickle cell disease (SCD) is one such issue. Originating from a genetic mutation which historically developed as a form of protection against malaria, SCD is a blood disorder which can cause pain, tiredness and fatigue, and has commonly been associated with individuals from African and Afro-Caribbean backgrounds. Yet it does not exclusively affect these groups. Individuals from Middle Eastern, southern European and Hispanic backgrounds have the potential to develop it. Overall, Barry and Yuill (2016) argue, those who are at risk are primarily individuals whose ancestry lies within a country where malaria was commonplace at one point. Although its origins lie within the genetic structure of an individual, from the evidence available it can be concluded that the actual distribution of SCD is, in fact, far more widespread among individuals from different ethnic backgrounds than has been commonly thought. It is inaccurate to suggest that it can be identified with one or only a handful of ethnic groups, as its prevalence cuts across a varying number of different peoples.

With SCD having been commonly associated with African and Afro-Caribbean individuals, this is an illustration of what Carter and Dyson (2011) describe as the ethnoisation of disease. This, they assert, refers to the popular association of a specific disease with one particular ethnicity, while conversely assuming that it does not impact upon others. As there is limited evidence that biology and genetics account for much of the variation in health status among ethnic groups, there exists little reason to believe that there are certain ethnic minority groups who are more prone to experience certain diseases simply as a result of their ethnicity.

4.8.2 Ethnicity and health: a complex picture

Efforts to understand the relationship between ethnicity and health are invariably complex. Nonetheless, it is possible to identify a broad picture. Evidence produced by Raleigh and Holmes (2021) illustrated the complexity of ethnic health inequalities; they argued that, in the UK, health inequalities exist between ethnic minorities and the ethnic majority population, as well as between ethnic minorities themselves. Drawing upon evidence from self-reported perceptions of their own health, Raleigh and Holmes (2021) argued that ethnic minority groups, in particular Pakistani and Bangladeshi individuals, are more likely to report long-term illness and poor health than White British population groups. Moreover, White Gypsy and Irish Traveller individuals reported the poorest health of all ethnic groups.

Focusing on specific aspects of health, Raleigh and Holmes (2021) identified some notable inequalities. In relation to maternal mortality, although the absolute numbers are relatively low, compared to white mothers, women from Black ethnic backgrounds were more than four times as likely to die during childbirth, with women from Asian backgrounds twice as likely. Additionally, Raleigh and Holmes (2021) found rates of infant mortality were greater among ethnic minorities. In examining why this was so varied among ethnic groups, however, poverty and deprivation were identified as significant, with a higher proportion of mothers from ethnic minority backgrounds living in poverty compared to white mothers. Deprivation, it was argued, could also account for the higher rates of childhood obesity among Black and Asian children. Among adults, it has been identified that those from South Asian groups consistently exhibit higher rates of cardiovascular disease compared with individuals from white backgrounds, as well as the national average. On the other hand, individuals from Black backgrounds have lower rates than the national average.

When examining the determinants of ethnic minority health, Raleigh and Holmes (2021) largely disregard smoking and alcohol, with levels of use largely lower among ethnic minorities compared to the white population. Furthermore, rates of physical activity vary among ethnic minorities, while, on average, ethnic minority individuals are less likely to eat the recommended portions of fruit and vegetables per day.

That health issues can disproportionately impact upon ethnic minorities was significantly illustrated during the Covid-19 pandemic of 2020–21. Among other studies illustrating similar evidence, Sze *et al.* (2020) argued that there was a clear correlation between ethnicity and Covid-19, with higher infection rates among Asian and Black ethnic minority communities in both the UK and the USA. Similarly, Khanijahani's (2021) analysis identified both higher infection rates and mortality levels as a consequence of Covid-19 among communities with large black ethnic minority populations in the USA. Moreover, Raleigh and Holmes (2021) argued that in the UK, during the first wave of Covid-19, ethic minority groups had higher rates of mortality than the white British population. A knee-jerk reaction to such evidence would be to try to identify the causes of increased ethnic minority susceptibility within biological and genetic explanations. However, the evidence for this has been, at best, negligible. In an effort to understand why ethnic minorities have a tendency to display poorer rates of health and wellbeing, we must look to social and economic factors.

4.8.3 Social and economic inequality and ethnicity

It has been common to try to explain health disparities among ethnic groups by reducing them to cultural factors, arguing that the origins of ethnic minority ill health are located within the cultural norms and values of the ethnic minority group, with any disadvantage being the result of their own practices and attitudes. This perspective, however, has been labelled as a 'blaming' approach, as it is the culture of the ethnic minority group which is considered at fault

(Nazroo, 2004). As with biological and genetic arguments, this approach ignores social and economic inequalities which contribute to health disparities.

In wealthy nations, including the UK, it is not uncommon for many ethnic minorities to live in conditions of social deprivation, experiencing poverty, low income and unemployment on a scale greater than the ethnic majority population. Recognising the relationship between socioeconomic status and health, Raleigh and Holmes (2021) argued that Asian and Black groups are more likely to live in a low income household than members of the white British population, overcrowding is higher among ethnic minority households, while unemployment in Pakistani, Bangladeshi and Black communities is roughly double the national average. From research conducted during the 1990s, Nazroo (2004) concluded that there was a strong relationship between socioeconomic status and the health of all ethnic minorities, as once the impact of socioeconomic status was removed, the risk of poor health was reduced. Evidence from the USA supported this, with both high income white and black populations displaying greater health than their lower income counterparts (Williams, 2012). Overall, the last quarter of a century has demonstrated that socioeconomic inequality is one of the principal reasons for health disparities experienced by ethnic minorities (Nazroo, 2010).

The consequence of economic inequality for ethnic minority health was illustrated with regard to Covid-19. In their analysis, Sze *et al.* (2020) asserted that a higher proportion of ethnic minorities in the USA were more likely to experience lower socioeconomic status, resulting in an increased chance of living within overcrowded households and sharing communal facilities, thus exacerbating the risk of contact with others who may potentially have had Covid-19. This was supported by Iacobucci (2020) in the UK, who argued that living conditions and occupation influenced rates of Covid-19 among ethnic minorities.

4.8.4 Discrimination and prejudice

Socioeconomic status undoubtedly has a significant impact on health; yet, when factors accounting for its impact are adjusted, there remain disparities of health between ethnic minorities and the ethnic majority populations. When the health status of ethnic minority and ethnic majority individuals within the same socioeconomic position are compared, ethnic minority individuals still display poorer health. As Nazroo (2004) argues, there exists another component of ethnicity which increases ethnic minorities' susceptibility to poor health; namely, discrimination and prejudice.

Racial prejudice in the UK towards ethnic minorities is very difficult to quantify, primarily due to reservations by individuals with regard to admitting to being prejudiced. One attempt illustrated in 2017 that 36% of the UK population described themselves as racially prejudiced to varying degrees (Kelley, Khan and Sharrock, 2017). Racial prejudice, both in terms of being a victim and the awareness that such attitudes exist, can have significant negative consequences for an individual's health, in particular their mental health (Annandale, 2014; Barry and Yuill, 2016).

Similarly, racially prejudiced attitudes can be embedded within the way society operates, with its social structures and institutions functioning in a racist manner. Thus, rather than just focusing on the actions of individuals, attention also needs to be drawn to social structures and institutions which operate in a discriminatory manner and which subsequently influence the actions and attitudes of those located within them. Institutional and structural discrimination can, at times, characterise both health and other governmental services which collaborate with the health sector. This can be exemplified in relation to mental health, where the institutional attitudes and practices of mental health services and the criminal justice system have been argued as contributing to some of the ethnic disparities identified in relation to mental illness.

ACTIVITY 4.11

In what ways do you think racism and discrimination can impact negatively upon an individual's health?

CHAPTER SUMMARY

- Health is not just a biological phenomenon, caused by the malfunctioning of the body and its biological system. Rather, health is as much a social phenomenon.
- Not everyone in society has an equal chance of experiencing good and poor health. The experience of good health is unevenly distributed in society. The result is a society characterised by health inequalities.
- There exist various social determinants of health which contribute to its uneven distribution among the population.
- As well as focusing upon medical interventions in order to promote positive health, it is important to understand that a fundamental component of a healthy population is a healthy society, one in which efforts are made to mitigate against those aspects of society which contribute to poor health.

FURTHER READING

Barry, A. and Yuill, C. (2016) *Understanding the Sociology of Health*, 4th edition. Sage.

Humber, L. (2019) *Vital Signs: the deadly costs of health inequality*. Pluto Press.

Walsh, M. (2018) *Key Topics in Social Sciences: an A–Z guide for student nurses*. Lantern Publishing.

White, K. (2017) *An Introduction to the Sociology of Health and Illness*, 3rd edition. Sage.

References

Annandale, E. (2014) *The Sociology of Health and Medicine: a critical introduction*, 2nd edition. Polity.

Barry, A. and Yuill, C. (2016) *Understanding the Sociology of Health*, 4th edition. Sage.

Bartley, M. (2016) *Health Inequality: an introduction to concepts, theories and methods*, 2nd edition. Polity.

Broom, D. (2012) 'Gender and health'. In Germov, J. (ed.) *Second Opinion: an introduction to health sociology*, 4th edition. Oxford University Press.

Carter, B. and Dyson, S.M. (2011) Territory, ancestry and descent: the politics of sickle cell disease. *Sociology*, **45**(6): 963–76.

Dahlgren, G. and Whitehead, M. (1991) *Policies and Strategies to Promote Social Equity in Health*. Institute for Futures Studies. Available at: https://core.ac.uk/download/pdf/6472456.pdf (accessed 22 November 2022).

Engels, F. (2009[1845]) *The Condition of the Working Class in England*. Oxford University Press.

Germov, J. (2012) 'Health sociology and the social model of health'. In Germov, J. (ed.) *Second Opinion: an Introduction to health sociology*, 4th edition. Oxford University Press.

Humber, L. (2019) *Vital Signs: the deadly costs of health inequality*. Pluto Press.

Iacobucci, G. (2020) Covid-19: increased risk among ethnic minorities is largely due to poverty and social disparities, review finds. *BMJ*, 371. Available at: www.bmj.com/content/371/bmj.m4099 (accessed 22 November 2022).

Karlsen, S. and Nazroo, J. (2000) 'Identity and structure: rethinking ethnic inequalities in health'. In Graham, H. (ed.) *Understanding Health Inequalities*. Open University Press.

Kelley, N., Khan, O. and Sharrock, S. (2017) *Racial Prejudice in Britain Today*. Available at: http://natcen.ac.uk/media/1488132/racial-prejudice-report_v4.pdf (accessed 22 November 2022).

Khanijahani, A. (2021) Racial, ethnic, and socioeconomic disparities in confirmed COVID-19 cases and deaths in the United States: a county-level analysis as of November 2020. *Ethnicity & Health*, **26**(1): 22–35.

Marmot, M. (2016) *The Health Gap: the challenge of an unequal world*. Bloomsbury.

Marmot, M., Allen, J., Boyce, T., Goldblatt, P. and Morrison, J. (2020) *Health Equity in England: the Marmot Review 10 years on*. Available at: www.health.org.uk/publications/reports/the-marmot-review-10-years-on or bit.ly/3SL8ECE (accessed 22 November 2022).

Matthews, D. (2019) Capitalism and mental health. *Monthly Review*, **70**(8): 49–62.

Morrall, P. (2009) *Sociology and Health: an introduction*, 2nd edition. Routledge.

Nazroo, J.Y. (2004) 'Genetic, cultural or socioeconomic vulnerability? Explaining ethnic inequalities in health'. In Bury, M. and Gabe, J. (eds) *The Sociology of Health and Illness: a reader*. Routledge.

Nazroo, J. (2010) 'Health and health care'. In Bloch, A. and Solomons, J. (eds) *Race and Ethnicity in the 21st Century*. Palgrave.

Nazroo, J., Edwards, A. and Brown, G. (1997) Gender differences in the onset of depression following a shared life event: a study of couples. *Psychological Medicine*, **27**: 9–19.

NMC (2018) *Standards of Proficiency for Nursing Associates.* Nursing and Midwifery Council.

ONS (2021) *Health State Life Expectancies by National Deprivation Deciles, England: 2017 to 2019.* Office for National Statistics. Available at: www.ons.gov.uk/peoplepopulationandcommunity/healthandsocialcare/healthinequalities/bulletins/healthstatelifeexpectanciesbyindexofmultipledeprivationimd/2017to2019#:~:text=DFLE%20at%20birth%20for%20females,in%20the%20least%20deprived%20areas or bit.ly/3KLFaCo (accessed 22 November 2022).

Public Health England (2021) *Caring as a Social Determinant of Health: findings from a rapid review of reviews and analysis of the GP Patient Survey.* Available at: https://assets.publishing.service.gov.uk/government/uploads/system/uploads/attachment_data/file/971115/Caring_as_a_social_determinant_report.pdf or bit.ly/3EIw1He (accessed 22 November 2022).

Raleigh, V. and Holmes, J. (2021) *The Health of People from Ethic Minority Groups in England.* The King's Fund. Available at: www.kingsfund.org.uk/publications/health-people-ethnic-minority-groups-england or bit.ly/3KHHQ49 (accessed 22 November 2022).

RSPH (2018) *Health on the High Street: running on empty 2018.* Royal Society for Public Health. Available at: www.rsph.org.uk/our-work/campaigns/health-on-the-high-street/2018.html or bit.ly/3kuxjyl (accessed 22 November 2021).

Sze, S., Pan, D., Nevill, C.R. *et al.* (2020) Ethnicity and clinical outcomes in COVID-19: a systematic review and meta-analysis. *The Lancet,* 29–30: Available at: www.thelancet.com/journals/eclinm/article/PIIS2589-5370(20)30374-6/fulltext (accessed 22 November 2022).

White, K. (2017) *An Introduction to the Sociology of Health and Illness,* 3rd edition. Sage.

WHO (2021a) *COVID-19 and the Social Determinants of Health and Health Equity: evidence brief.* World Health Organization. Available at: www.who.int/publications/i/item/9789240038387 (accessed 22 November 2022).

WHO (2021b) *Noncommunicable Diseases.* World Health Organization. Available at: www.who.int/news-room/fact-sheets/detail/noncommunicable-diseases (accessed 22 December 2022).

Williams, D. (2012) Miles to go before we sleep: racial inequalities in health. *Journal of Health and Social Behavior,* **53**(3): 279–95.

5 PSYCHOLOGY AND HEALTH
Graham Jones

This chapter relates to outcomes 1.6, 1.11, 2.2, 2.5, 2.6, 3.2 and 3.3 within the *Standards of Proficiency for Nursing Associates* (NMC, 2018).

LEARNING OUTCOMES

When you have completed this chapter you should be able to:
- Define the terms psychology and health psychology and describe the theories that underpin psychology.
- Explain the role of psychology within health and healthcare.
- Explore the role of psychology in explaining negative health behaviours.
- Outline the role that the 'locus of control' plays in determining health-related behaviours.

5.1 Introduction

This chapter provides an overview of the role of psychology within health and healthcare. The chapter initially defines psychology and health psychology, outlining their role in the healthcare environment. It goes on to consider how experiences can influence an individual's decision-making and health behaviours. The role that psychology plays in the management of health is discussed and an individual's locus of control is related to positive and negative health behaviours.

5.2 Psychology

The term 'psychology' is derived from the Greek word *psych*, which encapsulates the complexities associated with the mind, spirit and soul. Wilhelm Wundt, a professor at the University of Leipzig, is credited with creating the first psychology laboratory in 1880 where he exposed individuals to various stimuli, both auditory and visual, before exploring their perceptions of the experience.

Babu (2014, p. 4) defines psychology as the "scientific study of behaviour and mental processes". The application of psychology can support the nursing associate in delivering high quality, patient-centred care.

5.3 Psychology of health

Health is considered by the World Health Organization (WHO) as "a state of complete physical, mental and social wellbeing and not merely the absence of disease or infirmity" (WHO, 1948). Because this definition uses the term 'complete', it means that most people in society are 'unhealthy'. Think about how many people really are 'completely' healthy physically, psychologically, and socially at any one time. Consider an 85-year-old lady who has glaucoma, osteoporosis and type two diabetes. Despite her medical conditions the lady leads an active and fulfilling life participating in social activities which include playing bowls and being a member of her local pub quiz team. Accepting the WHO definition of health, she is unhealthy due to her medical conditions despite her ability to function independently, socially, physically and cognitively (Scholz *et al.*, 2014).

>> **Health psychology seeks to identify the various psychological factors which contribute to poor health.**

Health can be viewed as much more than the absence of disease. Perhaps a more relevant definition of health is provided by Sartorius (2006, p. 1) who defines health as "a state of balance, an equilibrium that an individual has established within himself and between himself and his social and physical environment". Huber *et al.* (2011) agree, viewing health as the "ability to adapt and self-manage". It is clear that defining health is complex and is linked to other variables, which leads to an exploration of the psychology associated with the term 'health'.

The psychology of health involves recognising the effect of biological, psychological and social factors on wellness and chronic illness (Hilton and Johnston, 2017). These factors include genetics, the environment, education, beliefs and behaviours and involve exploring the interaction between the body, mind and the environment.

Modern healthcare has moved away from simply treating illness and disease. There is now an emphasis on understanding the experiences of those affected and where possible preventing the onset of disease. The increase in chronic conditions such as cardiovascular disease, diabetes, obesity, chronic obstructive pulmonary disease (COPD) and cancers required a new public health approach, a movement that would limit chronic illness with preventative interventions and bring to the forefront the relevance of psychological health (Rawaf, 2018).

Health psychology seeks to identify the various psychological factors which contribute to poor health. It is fundamental to the role of the nursing associate as it allows a better understanding of people:

- How they handle illness
- Why some are able to adapt to lifestyle changes, e.g. a diabetic diet
- Why some engage in behaviours that are detrimental to health, e.g. smoking
- Why some are not able to follow health advice, e.g. taking regular medication.

5.4 Philosophy of psychology

In psychology, the theories of behaviourism, cognitivism and humanism are used to explain thoughts, emotions and behaviours (Muhajirah, 2020).

5.4.1 Behaviourism

Behaviourist principles state that the individual is susceptible to the stimulus of the environment and the behaviours they observe within that environment (Mukhalalati and Taylor, 2019). In simplistic terms, an individual's behaviour is learnt. If someone lives in a violent environment, that behaviour may be embraced by the individual throughout their life. The individual who is brought up in a household of smokers may learn and potentially adopt that behaviour. This can offer you as a nursing associate an appreciation of why some people engage in behaviours that are detrimental to their health.

5.4.2 Cognitivism

Cognitive psychologists look beyond behaviours. They believe that the decisions we make are an internal mental process. They focus on how information is received, organised, stored and retrieved; how it is processed. Individuals are believed to have and use the skills of inquiry and problem-solving (Aliakbari *et al.*, 2015) and can understand, interpret, process language and information, make sense of issues and therefore make appropriate healthy decisions. Factors that could alter this mental processing might include degenerative disease, social isolation, loneliness, stress, anxiety or depression by influencing cognitive clarity (Syrjämäka and Hietanen, 2019).

5.4.3 Humanism

Humanistic psychologists promote the individual's ability for self-actualisation, self-fulfilment, self-motivation and self-determination (Taylor and Hamdy, 2013). When applied to health, this theory stresses the importance of the person's individuality, free will and subjectivity. Humanism sees people as psychologically independent with consciousness and awareness, capable of taking control and making the right decisions based on their individual needs, whereas behaviourist theory implies that we are pawns of our environment. The humanistic approach seeks to understand and support the person by empowerment and advocacy.

5.4.4 Classical conditioning

For many people the term psychology brings to mind famous psychoanalysts and theorists like Sigmund Freud, John Bowlby, Jean Piaget, Erik Erikson and Ivan Pavlov who sought to explain the complexities of human development, thinking and behaviour. A detailed discussion of their work is beyond the remit of this chapter but their theories still inform today's thinking. For example, Ivan Pavlov coined the term 'classical conditioning' in terms of the learning process. He identified that dogs would salivate when presented with food, he referred to the food as an unconditional stimulus and the production of saliva the unconditional response. He then engaged in a level of manipulation by introducing what he described as the 'neutral' stimulus, a ringing bell. Every time Pavlov fed the dogs he would also introduce the neutral stimulus, the ringing of the bell. Over time the dogs would salivate upon hearing the bell, even in the absence of any food; they had been 'conditioned' to align the sound of the bell with food that in turn initiated a physiological response, salivation.

The principles of Pavlov's theory and classical conditioning can be applied to the behaviour of healthcare service users. An example is anticipatory nausea. Cancer patients undergoing chemotherapy will often experience nausea and vomiting as a physiological response to the treatment. They may subsequently need to attend the same hospital for a totally unrelated condition, but they may again experience nausea and vomiting; they are conditioned to associate the hospital with the condition (Rhodes and McDaniel, 2001). Similarly, studies have identified that former users of illicit drugs experience cravings when in a drug-related environment.

5.5 Approaches to health management

Historically, patient care was based on the biomedical model, outlined in *Chapter 4*. This approach was criticised as it viewed disease and illness as a biological process independent of psychological and social considerations (Engel, 1977). Engel believed that healthcare professionals needed to deliver patient-centred, individualised care that recognised the diverse physical, psychological and social factors experienced by those individuals.

This brought about the development of the biopsychosocial model which emphasises the relevance and influence of societal inequalities, education, employment, stress, anxiety, environment, poverty, housing, exclusion, culture, genetics, lifestyle and personal choice in determining an individual's health status (Borrell-Carrió, Suchman and Epstein, 2004), illustrated in *Figure 5.1*. The biopsychosocial model does not discard the relevance and importance of the biomedical approach.

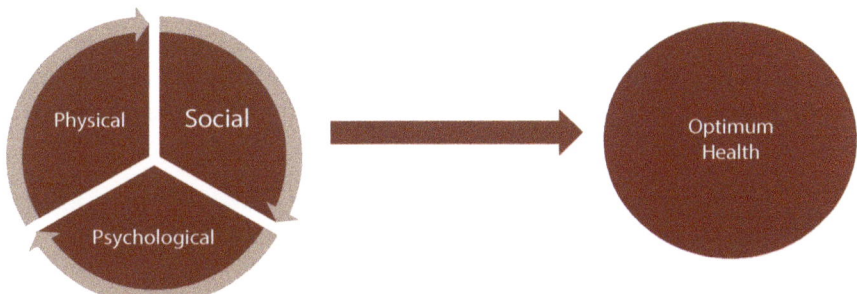

Figure 5.1 *The interaction of physical, psychological and social considerations contribute to optimum health.*

There is evidence to support the practical application of the biopsychosocial model. Research supports the association between lifestyle choices and illness: diet and obesity, smoking and lung disease, cancers and the environment, alcohol consumption and liver disease, unemployment and anxiety, heart disease and diet (McInerney, 2002). The physical presentation is brought about by the interplay of social and psychological experiences and equally the psychological presentation is a consequence of biological and social determinants (Abraham *et al.*, 2016).

RECAP

- Psychology is the study of human behaviour and the thoughts, feelings and motivations that lie behind behaviour.
- The psychology of health involves recognising the effect of biological, psychological and social factors on wellness and ill health.
- Health psychology affords the nursing associate a better understanding of people and how they respond to health issues.
- The three main theories used to explain thoughts, emotions and behaviours are behaviourism, cognitivism and humanism.
- The biopsychosocial model recognises the diverse physical, psychological and social factors experienced by individuals and can help to deliver patient-centred, individualised care.

5.6 Holism

Holism focuses on the importance of patient-centred care (PCC), illustrated in *Figure 5.2*, where the healthcare professional must work in close partnership with the patient to develop a therapeutic relationship based on the principles of care, compassion, respect and dignity (Peate, 2020). Nursing associates must ensure that their interactions with service users reflect these principles and that care is delivered in a collaborative manner. This supports individuals in developing the knowledge, skills and confidence to make decisions about their own health and healthcare (Health Foundation, 2016). In delivering PCC healthcare professionals interact with the individual, amalgamating the sum of the parts into a whole that includes the mind, body and soul (McMillan, Stanga and Van Sell, 2018).

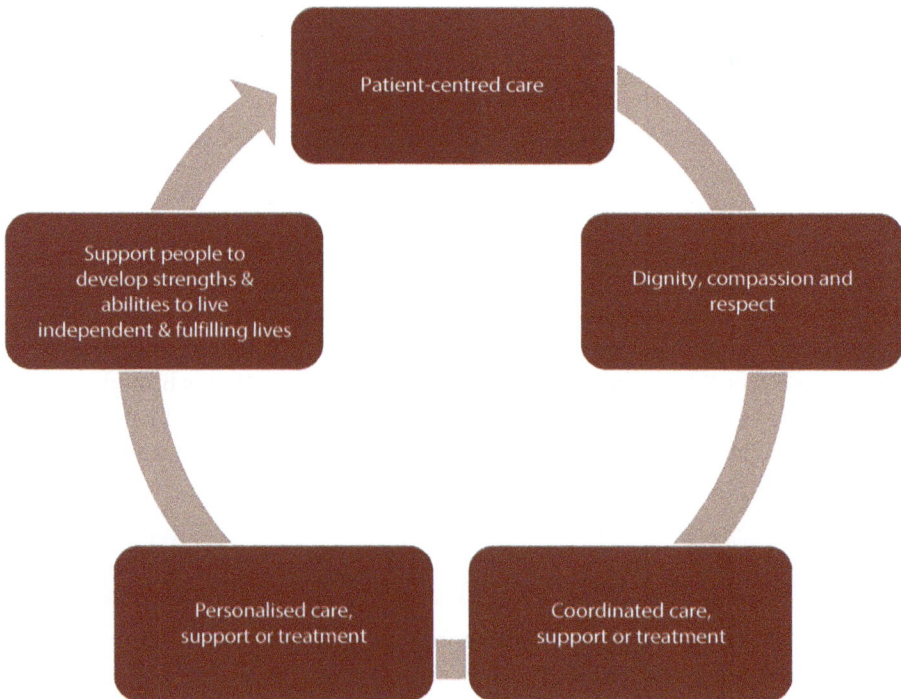

Figure 5.2 *The Health Foundation (2016) has identified a framework that comprises four principles of person-centred care.*

Advocates of holism or holistic health believe that the connected elements of the mind, body and spirit cannot be separated into individual parts (McMillan, Stanga and Van Sell, 2018). A disturbance in one part of the whole system, whether it is physical, psychological, spiritual or social, affects all other parts of the system. As a nursing associate, you need to be mindful of the impact that an individual's physical presentation may have on their psychological, social and spiritual health.

ACTIVITY 5.1

Consider the case study below.

In what ways do you think the biopsychosocial model is appropriate in this case?

CASE STUDY

You are a newly qualified nursing associate working on a regional spinal injuries unit. At the morning handover you are asked to care for Graham, a 25-year-old professional footballer who is married to Michelle. They have a one-year-old daughter, Sarah. Graham was admitted during the night through the emergency department following a road traffic collision. Following assessment and stabilisation Graham is diagnosed as having sustained a spinal cord injury (SCI) resulting in quadriplegia: having paralysis to his arms, hands, trunk, legs and feet.

Quadriplegia results from spinal cord injury (SCI) at the cervical level. The consequences of such an injury are catastrophic and life-changing. The impact on physical function may be obvious, but the significant impact on emotional and social wellbeing must also be recognised. Health-related quality of life for people with an SCI is significantly lower than for the general population (Tamplin *et al.*, 2014).

Graham could experience bladder and bowel dysfunction, coagulation dysfunction, chronic pain, pressure ulcers, chest and urinary tract infections, regulation of body temperature problems, loss of independence, loss of self-esteem, inability to earn an income, inability to have children and difficulties with developing intimate relationships, anxiety and depression. Anxiety and depression can result in withdrawal and poor communication (Warner, Ikkos and Gall, 2017) leading to secondary health issues such as alcohol and substance abuse. In turn, alcohol and substance abuse can have a detrimental impact on working life, relationships and social engagement. Using the biopsychosocial model and the concept of holism will ensure the care that Graham receives goes beyond his physical problems.

5.7 What makes us what we are?

Psychology and physiology are intricately connected (see *Figure 5.3*). The brain controls multiple functions that include maintaining homeostasis, thinking rationally, expressing emotions, problem-solving and learning. From this close relationship, there is an association between psychology and the mechanisms and progression of illness (Miller, Chen and Cole, 2009). Evidence links emotional wellbeing with the optimum functioning of the immune system, which protects the body from bacteria, viruses, parasites and fungi (Salovey *et al.*, 2000). Stress, anxiety and depression all impede a person's ability to combat infections, cancers and autoimmune disease (Cohen & Herbert, 1996).

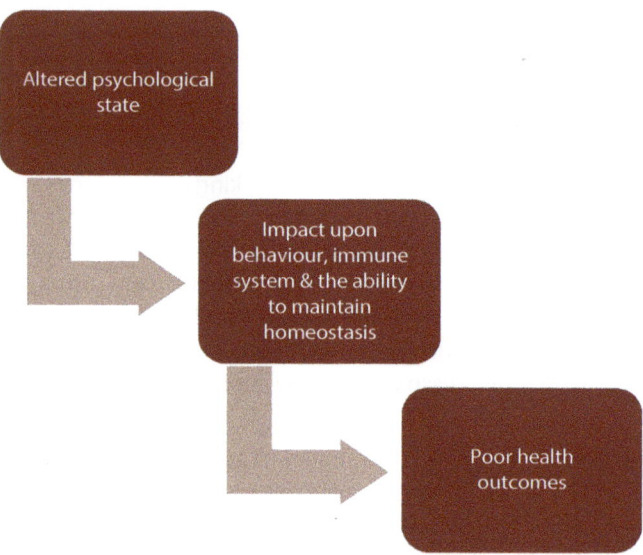

Figure 5.3 *The relationship between psychological and physiological states.*

Many factors contribute to poor physiological health and wellbeing, but it is important to appreciate the association with the individual's psychological status. This chapter identifies the links between human behaviour and health but it is worth remembering that an individual's psychological state can bring about alterations in their coping mechanisms and responses to stressors. For example, following bereavement an individual may experience grief, resulting in a poor sleep pattern. Their grief may lead to the development of detrimental health practices such as poor eating habits, smoking and excessive alcohol intake. These in turn can have a negative impact on the gastrointestinal system, respiratory system, liver function and memory (Cohen and Herbert, 1996). Relationship problems, financial problems and unemployment can all impact upon psychological wellbeing, which in turn impacts on physical wellbeing.

Psychological manifestations and modifiable lifestyle factors can all be seen as variables that contribute to quality of life, morbidity and indeed mortality. Our psychological 'self' influences the way we deal and cope with everyday stressors and subsequently how these daily stressors impact upon our physical health (De Hert *et al.*, 2011).

5.8 Behaviour

Despite an awareness of the detrimental impact that some actions have on our health and the potential to develop chronic illnesses as a result, many people fail to take the advice of public health officials. Our diet may be poor because we eat unhealthy food, we may drink too much alcohol at times, fail to take enough exercise and continue to smoke tobacco. Although there are significant efforts to promote more healthy lifestyles, globally unhealthy behaviours still lead to preventable diseases and cause substantial numbers of deaths (Busch and De Leeuw, 2014).

The drivers that direct individuals towards healthy choices, or indeed unhealthy choices, are multiple and complex. There are psychosocial, socioeconomic and biomedical determinants. Family dynamics, schooling, education, inequalities, peer groups, social deprivation, poverty, unemployment, and access to services all contribute to an individual's health status (Lazzeri *et al.*, 2014).

The links between psychosocial and socioeconomic status and suicide are well known. The Office of National Statistics (ONS, 2021) identified the suicide rate for men in England and Wales as 16 per 100,000 in 2021 (consistent with rates between 2018 and 2020) and a female suicide rate of 5.5 per 100,000 (consistent with rates between 2018 and 2020). Suicides were found to be higher in the lowest educational groups, the unemployed, those experiencing financial constraints, low family income, poverty, and those with a history of previous mental health problems (Näher, Rummel-Kluge and Hegerl, 2020). From a psychosocial perspective, a lack of meaningful family attachment has been found to increase not only suicidal thoughts but also suicidal behaviour. Some researchers believe that the family unit is the most significant factor in understanding suicide (Goldsmith *et al.*, 2002).

ACTIVITY 5.2

Think back to a time when you felt stressed. This might be when you were interviewed to become a trainee nursing associate, waiting to see a dentist, just before taking your driving test or sitting an examination at school.

Think about how you felt.

You may remember:
- Having a dry mouth
- Having butterflies in your stomach and not being able to face eating or drinking
- Feeling your heart beating faster and stronger than usual
- Feeling on edge.

Stress can be described as a situation that places an individual in a position where capacity is overcome by demand (Fletcher *et al.*, 2011). In modern life stress is often viewed in a negative light but it is an adaptive event and helps us to survive. Short-term acute stress helps to increase our alertness and performance (see *Table 5.1*). When we become frightened or anxious the adrenal medulla secretes adrenaline into the bloodstream in response to nerve impulses from the hypothalamus in the brain. This prepares the body for the fight or flight response, helping us to manage an urgent threat such as taking an examination or facing surgery. When the threat is over, the body returns to its usual state.

Table 5.1 *Acute stress*

Definition	An adaptive physiological, psychological and emotional reaction in response to a threatening situation
Causes	A perceived urgent threat such as injury, an emotional shock or impending surgery
Effects	The flight or fight response (also known as the alarm response or acute stress response) causing an increase in heart rate, blood pressure and blood flow to skeletal muscles, dilation of the airways to provide more oxygen to the bloodstream and muscles as well as an increase in the breakdown of glucagon to provide additional energy

Chronic, long-term stress (see *Table 5.2*) can have serious health consequences and may follow significant life events such as relationship breakdown, divorce, bereavement or the loss of a job. In chronic stress, the body response changes to the secretion of the hormones aldosterone and cortisol from the adrenal cortex. These raise the blood pressure and blood glucose as well as suppressing the immune system.

Table 5.2 *Chronic stress*

Definition	A long-term response triggered by life events leading to physical and psychological ill health
Causes	Varied life events, e.g. becoming seriously ill, bereavement, changing schools or moving house
Effects	In the immune system: a reduction in white blood cells may lead to increased infections. Damping down of the inflammatory response means that wounds take longer to heal.
	Other: increased blood glucose levels giving rise to tiredness, increased thirst and frequency of urination. Increased blood pressure. Headaches, mood swings, sleep disturbance, lack of concentration, memory problems, stomach upsets, diarrhoea, panic attacks, anxiety and depression.

We have all experienced some of the physiological effects of feeling stressed, such as a headache, churning stomach or insomnia, but stress also has an impact on our behaviour. Exposure to seemingly minor day-to-day, mundane events can cause anxiety and distress (Eck, Quick and Byrd-Bredbenner, 2021) and initiate negative behavioural changes. Some people may resort to a glass of wine after work to help deal with the daily stresses of a job and others might indulge in comfort eating when feeling stressed. Stress can also make us short-tempered, creating difficulties in our relationships with others. These are simplified examples of how behavioural change can be brought about by stressors. In reality, personality traits, gender, cognitive functioning, self-consciousness and situational factors (Sayette, 1999) will all play a role in determining the individual's response to stressful events.

Many behaviours detrimental to health can be modified with support and guidance. Cognitive theory implies that we are in control of our own destiny and make decisions to engage in healthy or unhealthy behaviours. The behaviourist view is that our behaviours are influenced by our environment. For example, a child who is not encouraged to brush their teeth and does not see their parents or carers clean their teeth may well adopt the very same behaviour.

Table 5.3 *Behaviours and potential impact on health*

Behaviour	Potential adverse health outcomes
Excessive alcohol use	Liver disease, cancers, gastrointestinal disease, infertility, sexual dysfunction, relationship issues, pancreatitis, diabetes, addiction & employment issues
Poor oral hygiene	Cardiovascular disease, periodontal disease, halitosis, dental caries, tooth loss, malnutrition & sepsis
Smoking	COPD, peripheral vascular disease, cancers, stroke, cardiovascular, immune system problems & addiction
Illicit drug use	Psychosis, hepatitis, HIV, depression, hallucinations, relationship issues, addiction, family breakdown & employment issues
Unhealthy diet	Obesity, heart disease, high blood cholesterol level & cancers
Sedentary lifestyle	Weight gain, hypertension, diabetes, cardiovascular disease & musculoskeletal problems

Each of the behaviours in *Table 5.3* is modifiable with appropriate encouragement, guidance and support from healthcare professionals. Individuals can be empowered to make behavioural change and healthier choices. Public health strategists have advocated the use of various models such as Tannahill's (2008) Education Model, the Health Belief Model, and the Transtheoretical (Stages of Change) Model to facilitate change in health behaviour.

ACTIVITY 5.3

Based on what you have read in this chapter, your life experience and any care experience you may have, write down a list of factors that can make someone more likely to have poor dental health.

Your list might contain some of these points:

- Hygiene: lack of good role models as a child to develop effective teeth cleaning and flossing habits.
- Diet: understanding personal diet and affordability and availability of sugar-rich foods.
- Provision of dental services: unable to register with a NHS dentist.
- Fluoride: lack of fluoride in local water supply and not using fluoride-based toothpaste.
- Financial: cost of treatment; some dental practices only offer care using an insurance-based model or 'pay per treatment' care. For most insurance-type services, teeth have to be in good condition before joining the scheme. Hourly paid workers may lose money if they take time off work to visit the dentist.

5.9 Locus of control

The amount of control that an individual has is a significant factor in how they respond to stressful events such as illness (*Figure 5.4*). Generally, people like to feel that they can make decisions and take actions that will influence a situation. Those that feel they have personal control over a situation are usually less stressed and considered to have an internal locus of control. People who think that their life is controlled by external forces such as luck or fate are said to have an external locus of control (Sarafino and Smith, 2016).

ACTIVITY 5.4

Although we are focusing on the locus of control in healthcare, it influences our beliefs about other areas of our lives. Think for a few minutes about how you might react to receiving a low grade in one of your assignments.

Would you consider:

- The amount of time that you spent gathering the evidence, reading about the subject, making notes and generally preparing for the assignment?
- Checking the examiner's feedback to see what you need to do to get a better grade next time?
- Taking any actions to improve your writing skills, such as revising your referencing technique using an online tutorial?

ACTIVITY 5.4 (continued)

Or would you be inclined to think that:

- You have wasted some of your time?
- Whatever you do seems to make no difference and you can't really change things?
- You aren't that good at essays/exams/referencing anyway?

Do you have an internal or external locus of control?

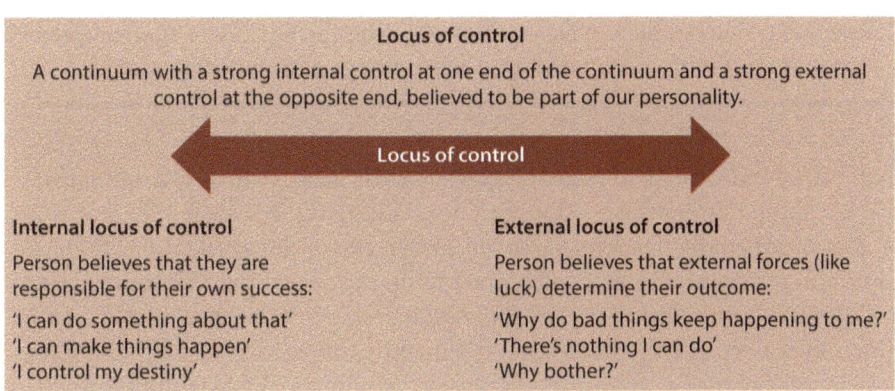

Figure 5.4 *Locus of control.*

Chronic illness and long-term conditions are features of modern societies where people live longer in old age. Teaching and supporting people with chronic illness to manage their condition through self-care is a fundamental part of enabling people to live independently. Educational programmes are a key part of this process.

Understanding how people view their locus of control can be useful when offering patient education programmes designed to support self-care and management to people with chronic health conditions (Wang *et al.*, 2022). Zhu *et al.* (2022) found that people with an internal locus of control managed their diabetes better, resulting in improved blood glucose control. Over time, this reduces the amount and severity of the complications associated with diabetes, leading to better health in the long term.

ACTIVITY 5.5

Prescribed medication is used to treat many conditions such as pain, swollen legs, infections and heart disease. Spend a few minutes thinking of reasons why someone may not take their medication as it was prescribed – make a list of these.

Your list might include:

The person may forget when to take the medication or run out of it. They may experience unpleasant side-effects such as constipation caused by codeine-based pain relief, and diarrhoea or thrush from antibiotics. They may find that the medication causes difficulties with their daily routine, for example taking diuretics may mean that a person can't go out to shop or go to appointments until later in the day, as they need to pass urine frequently.

Supporting individuals to make changes to their lives, such as changing their diet or taking regular medication, can be challenging. Between 30% and 50% of all prescribed medications are taken incorrectly or not at all (NICE, 2009). Promoting concordance extends beyond telling people to take their medicines and involves negotiating with the individual to understand their issues and difficulties when taking medication. Frequently the need to take medication long-term is part of a larger process where the individual is adapting to an altered life brought about by the diagnosis of illness. This experience can be similar to bereavement as it may include loss of future opportunities, functions or capacity and awareness that life changes may be permanent. An empathetic and person-centred approach can support concordance, but psychological adjustment to loss is not a rapid process (Allen, 2021).

ACTIVITY 5.6

To be able to register as a nursing associate, the NMC (2018) expects you to understand the principles of safe and effective administration and optimisation of medicines in accordance with local and national policies.

Write a list of any advice or actions that may help one of your patients achieve concordance in their prescribed medication.

Your list might include:

- Making sure they understand why the medication has been prescribed, the time of day it is to be taken and why
- If the medication is long-term they need to know who will issue the next prescription; if it is short-term, they need to know when the medication will stop

ACTIVITY 5.6 (continued)

- They may need to use a prescription and medication collection and delivery service so they have a continuous supply and know how to store their medication correctly
- Reminders / blister packs might need to be considered if the person has memory problems
- Some tamper-proof medicine containers are very difficult for weak or arthritic hands to open – discuss with the pharmacist. They must report difficulties to the prescriber as there may be alternative medication that can be taken instead.

5.10 Conclusion

The psychology of health is a multifaceted concept that involves exploration of the alignment between body, mind and environment. The people we meet as patients are a consequence of their early life experiences, cognitive development and social circumstances; a recognition of this helps the nursing associate understand why some embrace healthy lifestyles while others engage in activities that are detrimental to health.

Along with health promotion specialists, nursing associates have opportunities within their clinical role to support people to improve and maintain their mental, physical and behavioural health.

CHAPTER SUMMARY

- Psychology can help in understanding patients and support the nursing associate in delivering patient-centred care.
- Understanding the theoretical basis of health behaviours enables us to develop an awareness of why some individuals engage in behaviours that are serious threats to their health.
- Modern healthcare uses a biopsychosocial perspective in addressing the holistic needs of patients.
- The body, mind and spirit are inextricably linked and cannot be treated as separate body parts or in isolation.
- Stress can influence the manner in which we respond to life events and can induce health behaviours that are detrimental to health.
- Locus of control plays a significant role in determining how an individual reacts to health and illness.

FURTHER READING

Abraham, C. (2016) *Health Psychology*. Routledge.

Evans, D., Fathers, C.P. and Coutsaftiki, D. (2017) *Health Promotion and Public Health for Nursing Students*. Learning Matters.

Mooney, C.G. (2013) *Theories of Childhood: an introduction to Dewey, Montessori, Erikson, Piaget & Vygotsky*, 2nd edition. Redleaf Press.

Peate, I. (2021) *The Nursing Associate's Handbook of Clinical Skills* (Annexe A). Wiley-Blackwell.

Rodham, K. (2018) *Health Psychology*. Palgrave Macmillan.

References

Abraham, C., Conner, M., Jones, F. and O'Conner, D. (2016). *Health Psychology*, 2nd edition. Routledge.

Aliakbari, F., Parvin, N., Heidari, M. and Haghani, F. (2015) Learning theories application in nursing education. *Journal of Education & Health Promotion*, 4(2). Available at: https://pdfs.semanticscholar.org/ffe8/af0e4523cbaf723bb6fcbba9624c3d7e33fa.pdf?_ga=2.32576638.1557655881.1650026886-1496723769.1650026886 or bit.ly/3EHXqsv (accessed 6 December 2022).

Allen, L. (2021) Concordance and non-compliance: a psychological perspective. *Journal of Prescribing Practice*, 3(1): 28.

Babu, S. (2014) *Psychology for Nurses*. Elsevier.

Borrell-Carrió, F., Suchman, A.L. and Epstein, R.M. (2004) The biopsychosocial model 25 years later: principles, practice, and scientific inquiry. *Annals of Family Medicine*, 2(6): 576–582.

Busch, V. and De Leeuw, J.R. (2014) Unhealthy behaviours in adolescents: multi-behavioural associations with psychosocial problems. *International Journal of Behavioural Medicine*, 21(3): 439–446.

Cohen, S. and Herbert, T. (1996) Psychological factors and physical disease from the perspective of human psychoneuroimmunology. *Annual Review of Psychology*, 47: 113–42. Available at: www.researchgate.net/publication/14576696_HEALTH_PSYCHOLOGY_Psychological_Factors_and_Physical_Disease_from_the_Perspective_of_Human_Psychoneuroimmunology or bit.ly/3J0INDs (accessed 6 December 2022).

De Hert, M., Correll, C., Bobes, J. *et al.* (2011) Physical illness in patients with severe mental disorders. Prevalence, impact of medications and disparities in health care. *World Psychiatry*, 10(1): 52–77.

Eck, K.M., Quick, V. and Byrd-Bredbenner, C. (2021) Hassle exposure and reactivity links with obesogenic health behaviours. *American Journal of Health Behaviours*, 45(1): 161–173.

Engel, G.L. (1977) The need for a new medical model: a challenge for biomedicine. *Science*, 196(4286): 129–136.

Fletcher, B.C., Hanson, J., Page, N. and Pine, K.J. (2011) FIT – Do Something Different: a new behavioural program for sustained weight loss. *Swiss Journal of Psychology*, 70(1): 25–34.

Goldsmith, S.K., Pellmar, T.C., Kleinman, A.M. & Bunney, W.E. (eds) (2002) *Reducing Suicide: a national imperative*. National Academies Press.

Health Foundation (2016) *Person-centred Care Made Simple*. Available at: www.health.org.uk/publications/person-centred-care-made-simple or bit.ly/41EfYUK (accessed 6 December 2022).

Hilton, C.E. and Johnston, L.H. (2017) Health Psychology: it's not what you do, it's the way that you do it. *Health Psychology Open*, 4(2): 1–10.

Huber, M., Knottnerus, J.A., Green, L. *et al.* (2011) How should we define health? *BMJ*, 343: [d4163].

Lazzeri, G., Azzolini, E., Pammolli, A. *et al.* (2014) Factors associated with unhealthy behaviours and health outcomes: a cross-sectional study among Tuscan adolescents. *International Journal for Equity in Health*, **13**(1): 83. Available at: https://equityhealthj.biomedcentral.com/articles/10.1186/s12939-014-0083-5 (accessed 22 November 2022).

McInerney, S.J. (2002) What is a good doctor and how can we make one? Introducing the Biopsychosocial Model for good medicine and good doctors. *British Medical Journal*, **324**(1537). Available at: www.bmj.com/rapid-response/2011/10/29/introducing-biopsychosocial-model-good-medicine-and-good-doctors or bit.ly/2Q0n7di (accessed 6 December 2022).

McMillan, E., Stanga, N. and Van Sell, S.L. (2018) Holism: a concept analysis. *International Journal of Nursing & Clinical Practices*, **5**: 282. Available at: www.researchgate.net/publication/327109455_Holism_A_Concept_Analysis (accessed 6 December 2022).

Miller, G., Chen, E. and Cole, S. (2009) Health psychology: developing biologically plausible models linking the social world and physical health. *Annual Review of Psychology*, **60**: 501–24. Available at: www.annualreviews.org/doi/pdf/10.1146/annurev.psych.60.110707.163551 (accessed 6 December 2022).

Muhajirah, M. (2020) Basic of learning theory: (behaviourism, cognitivism, constructivism, and humanism). *International Journal of Asian Education*, **1**(1): 37–42.

Mukhalalati, B.A. and Taylor, A. (2019) Adult learning theories in context: a quick guide for healthcare professional educators. *Journal of Medical Education and Curricular Development*, **6**: 1–10. Available at: www.ncbi.nlm.nih.gov/pmc/articles/PMC6458658 (accessed 6 December 2022).

Näher, A-F., Rummel-Kluge, C. and Hegerl, U. (2020) Associations of suicide rates with socioeconomic status and social isolation: findings from longitudinal register and census data. *Frontiers in Psychiatry*, **10**: 898. Available at: www.ncbi.nlm.nih.gov/pmc/articles/PMC6971176 (accessed 6 December 2022).

NICE (2009) *Medicines Adherence: involving patients in decisions about prescribed medicines and supporting adherence*. Clinical guideline [CG76]. National Institute for Health and Care Excellence. Available at: https://www.nice.org.uk/guidance/cg76 (accessed 6 December 2022).

NMC (2018) *Standards of Proficiency for Nursing Associates*. Nursing and Midwifery Council. Available at: www.nmc.org.uk/standards/standards-for-nursing-associates/standards-of-proficiency-for-nursing-associates or bit.ly/3J0v4MK (accessed 6 December 2022).

ONS (2021) *Suicides in England and Wales: 2021 Registrations*. Office of National Statistics. Available at: www.ons.gov.uk/peoplepopulationandcommunity/birthsdeathsandmarriages/deaths/bulletins/suicidesintheunitedkingdom/2021registrations or bit.ly/3EMg6r4 (accessed 22 December 2022).

Peate, I. (2020) *Alexander's Nursing Practice: hospital and home*, 5th edition. Elsevier.

Rawaf, S. (2018) A proactive general practice: integrating public health into primary care. *Journal of Primary Care*, **10**(2): 17–18.

Rhodes, V. A. and McDaniel, R.W. (2001) Nausea, vomiting & retching: complex problems in palliative care. *Cancer Journal for Clinicians*, **2001**(51): 232–248. Available at: https://acsjournals.onlinelibrary.wiley.com/doi/pdfdirect/10.3322/canjclin.51.4.232 or bit.ly/3Y4Yuh6 (accessed 6 December 2022).

Salovey, P., Rothman, A.J., Detweiler, J.B. and Steward, W.T. (2000) Emotional states and physical health. *American Psychologist*, **55**(1): 110–121.

Sarafino, E.P. and Smith, T.W (2016) *Health Psychology: biopsychosocial interactions*, 9th edition. Wiley.

Sartorius, N. (2006) The meanings of health and its promotion. *Croat Med Journal*, **47**(4): 662–664.

Sayette, M.A. (1999) Does drinking reduce stress? *Alcohol Research & Health*, **23**(4): 250–255.

Scholz, U., König, C., Eicher, S. and Martin, M. (2014) Stabilisation of health as the centre point of a health psychology of ageing. *Psychology & Health*, **30**(6): 732–749.

Syrjämäki, A.H. and Hietanen, J.K. (2019) The effects of social exclusion on processing of social information – a cognitive psychology perspective. *British Journal of Social Psychology*, **58**(3): 730–748.

Tamplin, J., Baker, F.A., Grocke, D. and Berlowitz, D.J. (2014) Thematic analysis of the experience of group music therapy for people with chronic quadriplegia. *Top Spinal Cord Injury Rehabilitation*, **20**(3): 236–247.

Tannahill, A. (2008) Health promotion: the Tannahill model revisited. *Public Health*, **122**(12): 1387–91.

Taylor, D.C.M. and Hamdy, H. (2013) Adult learning theories: implications for learning and teaching in medical education: AMEE Guide No. 83. *Medical Teaching*, **2013**(35): 1561–1572.

Wang, R., Zhou, C., Wu, Y. *et al.* (2022) Patient empowerment and self-management behaviour of chronic disease patients: a moderated mediation model of self-efficacy and health locus of control. *Journal of Advanced Nursing*, **78**(4): 1055–1065. Available at: https://doi.org/10.1111/jan.15077 (accessed 6 December 2022).

Warner, N., Ikkos, G. and Gall, A. (2017) Spinal cord injury rehabilitation and mental health, SCReaM. *Spinal Cord*, **55**(3): 307–313.

WHO (1948) 'Constitution of the World Health Organization'. In: *World Health Organization: Basic documents*, 49th edition. World Health Organization. Available at: https://apps.who.int/gb/bd/pdf_files/BD_49th-en.pdf (accessed 6 December 2022).

Zhu, L., Shi, Q., Zeng, Y. et al. (2022) Use of health locus of control on self-management and HbA1c in patients with type 2 diabetes. Nursing Open, 9(2): 1028–1039. Available at: https://doi.org/10.1002/nop2.1140 (accessed 6 December 2022).

PUBLIC HEALTH AND HEALTH PROMOTION

Anneyce Knight

This chapter relates to outcomes 2.1 and 2.2 within the *Standards of Proficiency for Nursing Associates* (NMC, 2018a).

> ### LEARNING OUTCOMES
>
> When you have completed this chapter you should be able to:
> - Identify why public health and health promotion are relevant to your role as a nursing associate.
> - Define what public health and health promotion are.
> - Outline the historical context of public health and health promotion.
> - Explain the structure and priorities for public health in England.
> - Demonstrate an understanding of some key theories used to deliver successful health promotion.

6.1 Introduction

This chapter provides a broad overview of public health and health promotion that builds on the previous two chapters on society and health and psychology and health. The chapter begins by explaining why public health and health promotion are relevant and important to your role as a nursing associate. The historical context of both public health and health promotion are summarised and the roles of the Office for Health Improvement and Disparities, and the UK Health Security Agency, are also outlined. National and international public health priorities are presented, including a discussion of the NHS Long Term Plan (NHS, 2019). An explanation of health promotion is provided, followed by a summary of some theories related to developing health literacy and promoting health. By the end of this chapter you will understand the relationship between public health and health promotion, how they are essential to the promotion of health and the prevention of ill health, and improving health outcomes and addressing health inequalities.

105

6.2 Why are public health and health promotion relevant to my role as a nursing associate?

This is probably the first question you are asking yourself as you begin to read this chapter. The Nursing and Midwifery Council (NMC) (2018a) *Standards of Proficiency for Nursing Associates*, which the programme you are on complies with, states in Platform 2 (Promoting health and preventing ill health) that:

> *"Nursing associates play a role in supporting people to improve and maintain their mental, physical, behavioural health and wellbeing. They are actively involved in the prevention of and protection against disease and ill health, and engage in public health, community development, and in the reduction of health inequalities." (NMC, 2018a, p. 7).*

This is then broken down into nine areas which set out the knowledge and skills you need as a registered nursing associate for your role in health promotion, health protection and the prevention of ill health (NMC, 2018a).

ACTIVITY 6.1

Read page 6 of the NMC (2018a) *Standards of Proficiency for Nursing Associates* available at: www.nmc.org.uk/standards/standards-for-nursing-associates/standards-of-proficiency-for-nursing-associates or bit.ly/3GfXTDI and familiarise yourself with the nine proficiencies.

Which of the proficiencies do you feel confident in your knowledge and skills already?

This activity also relates to *Activity 6.9* at the end of the chapter.

Furthermore, *The Code: professional standards of practice and behaviour for nurses, midwives and nursing associates* (NMC, 2018b) (henceforth referred to as *The Code*) explains that in your role as a trainee nursing associate, and later as a registered nursing associate, you must:

> *"2.2 recognise and respect the contribution that people can make to their own health and wellbeing*
>
> *2.3 encourage and empower people to share decisions about their treatment and care*
>
> *3.1 pay special attention to promoting wellbeing, preventing ill health and meeting the changing health and care needs of people during all life stages*
>
> *3.3 act in partnership with those receiving care, helping them to access relevant health and social care, information and support when they need it."*

Both the NMC Standards (2018a) and *The Code* (NMC, 2018b) emphasise that the knowledge and skills related to public health and health promotion are a very important part of your everyday professional practice and delivery of care. Helping to prevent ill health, keeping people healthy and addressing health inequalities are as important as providing clinical nursing care for our service users/patients and their carers/families.

6.3 What is public health?

The four devolved nations of the UK have their own public health organisations – Public Health Scotland (PHS), Public Health Wales (PHW), Public Health Agency in Northern Ireland (PHANI) and, until September 2021, Public Health England (PHE). From 1 October

>> **The public health bodies of the four nations of the UK aim to protect and improve the health and wellbeing of the population.**

2021, the health improvement and public health work of PHE was transferred to the Office for Health Improvement and Disparities (OHID), NHS Digital, NHS England and NHS Improvements. PHE's health protection functions were moved to the United Kingdom Health Security Agency (UKHSA). These organisations aim to protect and improve the health and wellbeing of their nation's population and reduce health inequalities. Although each nation will have its own strategies and priorities to meet their population needs, they all have the common aim of protecting the health of the public and for PHS, PHW, PHANI this will continue to include improving health.

The Wanless (2004) definition of public health is:

"the science and art of preventing disease, prolonging life and promoting health, through organised efforts and informed choices of society, organisations, public and private, communities and individuals."

This expands the definition made by Acheson (1988), the definition used by the World Health Organization (WHO), which states that public health is the *"art and science of preventing disease, prolonging life and promoting health through the organized efforts of society"* (Acheson, 1988; WHO Regional Office for Europe, 2020).

ACTIVITY 6.2

What are the similarities and differences between the Wanless and Acheson / WHO definitions of public health?

It can be seen that public health not only involves protecting and promoting healthier lifestyles with individuals, families, communities and society as a whole, but also involves many other factors. These include (but not exclusively) research; collecting data; advising the NHS, the public, government and local government; providing and sharing information; preventing public health emergencies and responding to them and other challenges as required (consider Covid-19) (PHE, 2020).

6.4 History of public health

The first formal welfare interventions were provided ad hoc at local (parish) level by churches or religious orders; for example, by providing alms in the form of ale and bread. The Elizabethan Poor Laws of 1601 formalised this provision by seeking to address the health and welfare issues for the 'deserving' poor, which included those who were able-bodied but unable to work because they were ill or disabled, or those deemed to be too old. Others were seen as 'non-deserving' and therefore did not receive assistance. The legislation was amended with the Poor Law Amendment Act of 1834, which provided an institutionalised solution where help for the poor would only be provided in workhouses. The links we now understand between poverty, employment, housing and health were not understood then.

>> **Edwin Chadwick demonstrated that there were links between people's living conditions, their health and the spread of disease.**

Edwin Chadwick (1800–90) strove to reform the Poor Laws to improve the health of the population and is seen as the person who founded the public health movement. He investigated and published findings on *The Sanitary Conditions of the Labouring Population* in 1842. The evidence-based conclusions he came to demonstrated that there were links between this population's living conditions, their health and the spread of disease. He identified that people needed access to clean water, suitable drainage and the removal of refuse. This was the beginning of science informing public health interventions and initiating an awareness of what we now understand, i.e. that these are social determinants that affect health.

Later, in 1854, John Snow mapped an outbreak of cholera in London and, again using an evidence-based approach, traced the outbreak back to one water pump from which all those who had contracted the disease had drawn their water. This contributed to the understanding of how disease was spread. He is seen as the founder of epidemiology (understanding the incidence and spread of diseases and measures that could be used to control them).

The first Public Health Act was made by Parliament in 1848. The equivalent of today's local government authorities were made responsible for many public services including drainage and supplying clean water. This legislation, together with Victorian engineering innovations such as the sewerage system that Joseph Bazalgette designed for London, contributed to reducing the spread of diseases. Undoubtedly, clean water and sanitation have been, and continue to be worldwide, a major contributor to improving health and reducing the incidence of people dying at an earlier age than expected.

Further legislation that contributed to the continuing improvement in the health of the population came as a result of William Beveridge's Report on Social Insurance and Allied Services, published during the Second World War in 1942 (Parliament UK, 2020). He focused on addressing the 'five evils' which he saw in society: Want, Disease, Idleness, Ignorance and Squalor. This resulted in the welfare state that we know today. The National Health Service Act (1946) led to the birth of the NHS on 5 July 1948, the aim of which was to focus on eliminating all diseases. Other legislation included the Town and Country Planning Act (1947) which led to the demolition of slum housing and new homes being built, and the Education Act (1944) which meant that for the first time all children had access to free education up to the age of 15.

Many other factors have also contributed to the improvement in the UK population's health. These include:

- Therapeutics, such as the development of new medicines and antibiotics
- Legislation relating to the production of food (e.g. Food Standards Act, 1999) and banning smoking in public places (Health Act, 2006)
- Disease prevention and eradication using immunisation and vaccination programmes
- Screening programmes
- Improved diagnostics
- Increased understanding of lifestyle factors, such as smoking and alcohol which affect health
- Health and safety legislation relating to the workplace
- Since the late 1970s, the recognition of the importance of health promotion and personal responsibility to prevent ill health.

From this brief overview of the historical development of public health within the UK we can see there are many influences that have contributed to improving the population's health, increasing individual life expectancy and enhancing their quality of life.

6.5 The structure of English public health

As nursing associate roles are exclusive to NHS England, we will be focusing on the structure of public health in England only.

6.5.1 Office for Health Improvement and Disparities (OHID)

The OHID was established on 1 October 2021 as part of the Department for Health and Social Care, replacing Public Health England. Public Health England had a huge remit and possibly because of the significant health disparities found within some communities, exposed during the Covid-19 pandemic, the government decided that urgent action needed to be taken. The timing and nature of the changes drew considerable criticism.

The social and economic conditions in which we live play a substantial role in determining the quality of health and life expectancy. OHID is expected to address health inequalities by implementing preventative programmes targeting factors that damage health and shorten life, such as tobacco, obesity, alcohol and recreational drug use. Programmes will transcend local and central government, the NHS and society and will:

"focus on improving the nation's health so that everyone can expect to live more of life in good health, and on levelling up health disparities to break the link between background and prospects for a healthy life".

OHID will:
- "identify and address health disparities, focusing on those groups and areas where health inequalities have greatest effect
- take action on the biggest preventable risk factors for ill health and premature death including tobacco, obesity and harmful use of alcohol and drugs
- work with the NHS and local government to improve access to the services which detect and act on health risks and conditions, as early as possible
- develop strong partnerships across government, communities, industry and employers, to act on the wider factors that contribute to people's health, such as work, housing and education
- drive innovation in health improvement, harnessing the best of technology, analytics, and innovations in policy and delivery, to help."

For more information on the role of the OHID and its remit, visit: www.gov.uk/government/organisations/office-for-health-improvement-and-disparities/about or bit.ly/3IERhPc

6.5.2 UK Health Security Agency

The UKHSA became fully operational on 1 October 2021, building on the infrastructure developed in response to the Covid-19 pandemic with a focus on health protection and security. Initially named the National Institute for Health Protection (NIHP), it brought together PHE, NHS Test and Trace and the Joint Biosecurity Centre (JBC) under one leadership team (Gov.UK, 2020).

The responsibilities of UKHSA are:
1. Protecting every member of every community from the impact of infectious diseases, chemical, biological, radiological and nuclear incidents and other health threats

2. Providing intellectual, scientific and operational leadership at national and local level, as well as on the global stage, to make the nation's health secure. (Gov.UK, 2021)

6.5.3 The role of local authorities in public health

Local government authorities (e.g. county councils, unitary authorities, Metropolitan Boroughs and London Boroughs) [henceforth all referred to as local authorities] have the responsibility for promoting the health of their local population and planning for their needs. This responsibility moved from the NHS to local authorities on 1 April 2013. Their other responsibilities include education, social care, local economic development and housing, which as we are aware are social determinants of health (see *Chapter 4*). They aim to work in partnership with a number of government agencies (e.g. OHID) and private organisations (e.g. high street chemists), as well as focusing on prevention and ensuring health is embedded in all local authority policies. Each local authority has a Director of Public Health who works with their public health team. The Director of Public Health is a member of their local Health and Wellbeing Board and, as part of their role, produces an annual report on the health of their community's population.

Each local area (locality) produces a Joint Strategic Needs Assessment (JSNA) which has been the responsibility of the local Health and Wellbeing Board since the Health and Social Care Act of 2012. The JSNA

>> **Local authorities have responsibility for promoting the health of their local population.**

involves not just the local authority and their public health department but also organisations such as the local NHS Trusts (mental health, community and acute), community organisations, the voluntary sector (non-governmental organisations) and service users all working together in partnership. The evidence identifies and assesses the health and social care needs of their local population. Based on this evidence, plans are drawn up to address local health inequalities, improve life expectancy and health outcomes. These plans also inform the decisions about which specific health, wellbeing and social care services need to be bought (commissioned) to achieve this.

Although local authorities can decide on their own priorities and services, they do fund and commission preventative health services. These can include smoking cessation, drug and alcohol services and sexual health services; in addition they provide early years support for children (NHS, 2019). Local authorities ensure the plans they put in place to promote the health of their population meet the requirements of the NHS Long Term Plan (NHS, 2019) and local specific needs.

ACTIVITY 6.3

Search the internet and find the annual public health report for the area in which you are undertaking your trainee nursing associate programme.
- What initiatives have been implemented to improve the health of this population?
- How could you be involved in these initiatives?

6.6 World Health Organization and global public health

The global Covid-19 pandemic which started in 2019 demonstrates the speed at which a communicable disease can travel across international borders. It also shows us how a public health issue can impact on our own national economy and daily way of living with the public health measures taken to protect the whole population. It has also highlighted other factors such as our global economic interdependency and international connectivity/travelling and illustrates how we live in a global society. Globalisation *"refers to a range of processes that have the effect of bringing dispersed populations into closer contact, creating a single, integrated community of interest or independent society"* (Walsh, 2018, p. 78).

WHO, as a worldwide organisation, aims to "promote health, keep the world safe, and serve the vulnerable" (WHO, 2020). In its 2007 report, *The World Health Report 2007 – A Safer Future: global public health security in the 21st century* it identifies the need for global health security, which requires individual countries to work together. Collaborating in this way will identify risks to health and provide shared solutions for common public health challenges such as Covid-19 and the search for treatments and vaccines. Across the WHO European Region, including the UK, common challenges include (WHO Regional Office for Europe, 2020):
- "economic crisis
- widening [health] inequalities
- ageing population
- increasing levels of chronic disease
- migration and urbanization
- environmental damage and climate change".

6.7 The NHS Long Term Plan and national public health priorities

The NHS Long Term Plan (NHS, 2019) sets out a structured and systematic approach for the NHS to act on preventing ill health and addressing health inequalities. It acknowledges that this is not the exclusive role of the NHS, as prevention also involves local authorities, individuals, communities, national government and business and voluntary sectors. The Plan builds on the progress made from the *NHS England Five Year Forward View* report published in 2014 which recommended changes to the healthcare system and provided an emphasis on preventing ill health and *Next Steps on the NHS Five Year Forward View* (NHS England, 2014; NHS England, 2017).

The NHS Long Term Plan recognises that there will be future demands on the NHS to help people to stay healthier for longer. It has the specific aim of people gaining an extra five years of healthy life expectancy by 2035 (NHS, 2019). The demands identified include our ageing population, unmet health needs (e.g. long waiting lists for treatment, access to district nursing care or young people's mental health services) and innovation in diagnostics and treatments. Ensuring that the right care is delivered at the right time is, and will be, vital. Emphasis is also placed on 'upstream prevention' whereby self-management by service users/ patients of their disease, especially those with long-term health conditions, can reduce both their symptoms and admission to hospital (NHS, 2019, p. 33). This would not only enhance service users'/patients' quality of life but would also reduce the financial demand on the NHS. The service user/patient, and their carer and volunteers, need to be supported and empowered if self-management is to be successful (NHS, 2019).

The NHS Long Term Plan cites the Global Burden of Disease (GBD) 2018 study which identifies the top five risk factors that cause premature (early) death in the UK (Steel *et al.*, 2018). These are:

- Smoking
- Poor diet
- High blood pressure
- Obesity
- Alcohol and drug use.

(NHS, 2019, p. 33).

The GBD (2018) study also acknowledges that other factors such as air pollution, lack of exercise and antimicrobial resistance are also important risk factors. These public health concerns influence the NHS's prevention strategy. The Long Term Plan (NHS, 2019) also addresses other public health issues including *"a strong start in life for children and young people"* and *"better care for major health conditions"* as well as discussing workforce requirements and use of digital technologies.

This Plan highlights that:

> *"Every 24 hours, the NHS comes into contact with over a million people at moments in their lives that bring home the personal impact of ill health. It sets out practical action to do more to use these contacts as positive opportunities to help people improve their health" (NHS, 2019, p. 34).*

As a nursing associate (trainee or registered) your caring role brings you into direct contact with many people every day, whether in hospital or community settings. This provides you with daily opportunities to use health promotion strategies to enable your service users/patients to self-manage their health and for their carers/families to also improve their health (NMC, 2018b).

> **RECAP**
>
> - Public health is relevant to your role, as nursing associates are expected to engage in public health, community development and the reduction of health inequalities.
> - Public health has been defined as "the science and art of preventing disease, prolonging life and promoting health, through organised efforts and informed choices of society, organisations, public and private, communities and individuals."

6.8 What is health promotion?

Understanding health promotion is important, as it is part of your role as a trainee and registered nursing associate. The Ottawa Charter (WHO, 1986) defines it thus:

> *"Health promotion is the process of enabling people to increase control over, and to improve, their health. To reach a state of complete physical, mental and social wellbeing, an individual or group must be able to identify and to realize aspirations, to satisfy needs, and to change or cope with the environment. Health is, therefore, seen as a resource for everyday life, not the objective of living. Health is a positive concept emphasizing social and personal resources, as well as physical capacities. Therefore, health promotion is not just the responsibility of the health sector but goes beyond healthy life-styles to wellbeing."*

This definition of health promotion is holistic, as it identifies the importance of physical, mental and social aspects of health and wellbeing. It acknowledges that health is important for an individual to lead their life in the way they wish to and includes their families and communities. It emphasises that the empowerment (discussed later in this chapter) of individuals and communities is essential to improving their health.

Naidoo and Wills (2016) also place an emphasis on empowerment in their definition:

> *"Health promotion is a range of activities and interventions to enable people to take greater control over their health. Activities may be directed at individuals, families, communities or whole populations." (ibid., p. 125).*

The UK National Institute for Health and Care Excellence (NICE) provides a recent definition stating that health promotion is:

"... giving people the information or resources they need to improve their health. As well as improving people's skills and capabilities, it can also involve changing the social and environmental conditions and systems that affect health." (NICE, 2019).

Sometimes people confuse giving information or resources as the total extent of health promotion; this is health education, which is only one approach to health promotion.

6.9 History of health promotion

Today's understanding of health promotion relates back to when the term was first used at WHO's International Conference on Primary Health Care at Alma-Ata (present-day Almaty in Kazakhstan) in 1978 (Naidoo and Wills, 2016). At this conference the call was made *"for urgent action by all governments, all health and development workers, and the world community to protect and promote the health of all the people of the world"* (WHO, 1978, p. 1). At the first International Conference on Health Promotion in Ottawa, Canada, in 1986, what is known as the Ottawa Charter for action to achieve Health for All by 2000 was launched and their definition for health promotion adopted worldwide (WHO, 2009).

The second International Conference on Health Promotion in Adelaide (Australia), in 1988, built on the recommendations of Alma-Ata and Ottawa with calls for healthy public policy (WHO, 2009). This was

>> **The Alma-Ata Declaration and the Ottawa Charter are two milestones in the field of public health.**

followed in 1991 by the Third International Conference on Health Promotion in Sundsvall, Sweden which focused on Supportive Environments for Health (WHO, 2009). The Fourth International Conference (1997) in Jakarta, Indonesia, was entitled 'New Players for a New Era – leading health promotion into the 21st century' where the Jakarta declaration for action in health promotion was set for the next century (WHO, 2009). A fifth international conference followed in Mexico in 2000 and a sixth in Bangkok, Thailand, in 2005, where the Bangkok Charter for Health in a globalised world was launched. It upheld the importance of *"policies and partnerships to empower communities and to improve health and health equality, [which] should be at the centre of global and national development"* (WHO, 2006, p. 24). Subsequent conferences have been held in Nairobi, Kenya (2009), Helsinki, Finland (2013) and Shanghai, China (2016), the latter having a specific focus on the United Nations' Sustainable Development Goals (SDGs).

ACTIVITY 6.4

Read the 17 SDGs available at: www.un.org/sustainabledevelopment/sustainable-development-goals or bit.ly/3U8g6Z0

Goal 3 is to *"Ensure healthy lives and promote wellbeing for all at all ages."* Identify one health promotion activity you have either seen in your placement area, or been involved in, that would contribute to this goal.

From this brief historical context of health promotion, you can see the global momentum that has developed around health promotion since the concept emerged in the late 1970s/early 1980s.

6.10 The importance of the Ottawa Charter

The Ottawa Charter still informs health promotion practice today. It named three fundamental principles to delivering successful health promotion and improving everyone's health, while taking into account specific individual needs which will differ based on their "social, cultural and economic systems" (WHO, 1986). These three principles are:

Advocate

The Charter identified that good health is important for all aspects of life (e.g. work, quality of life) and any health promotion should advocate a holistic approach and address factors that can impact on this (e.g. economic, political or biological factors).

Enable

Health promotion should aim to reduce inequalities in health (see *Chapter 4*), support equal opportunities and ensure everyone can achieve their best possible health. This includes the chance to access information, develop life skills and be able to make healthy choices.

Mediate

Health promotion needs coordinated action at the micro level (e.g. your actions as a nursing associate and those of your health and social care colleagues, individuals, families and communities) and the macro level (e.g. local and national governments, non-governmental/voluntary organisations, industry, and the media) (WHO, 1986).

ACTIVITY 6.5

Read more about these principles and the five health promotion action areas which are set out in the Ottawa Charter available at: www.who.int/healthpromotion/conferences/previous/ottawa/en or bit.ly/41LLEHM

Which of the five health promotion action areas is most relevant to your role as a nursing associate and why?

6.11 Developing health literacy

From reading the five health promotion action areas in *Activity 6.5* you will have seen that emphasis is placed in health promotion on empowering people and enabling them to develop personal strategies and skills to make their health lifestyle choices throughout their lifespan (WHO, 1986). This is associated with health literacy, which can be defined thus:

"[it]... implies the achievement of a level of knowledge, personal skills and confidence to take action to improve personal and community health by changing personal lifestyles and living conditions. Thus, health literacy means more than being able to read pamphlets and make appointments. By improving people's access to health information, and their capacity to use it effectively, health literacy is critical to empowerment." (WHO, 1998).

6.11.1 Health education

Naidoo and Wills (2016, p. 57) define health education as *"activities to facilitate health related learning and behaviour change"* and state that it is an integral part of developing health literacy. Prior to the Ottawa Charter, health education was the approach used. Individuals were told how to prevent disease with information given to them and they were often made to feel guilty about their health choices in order to coerce them into changing their health behaviour (Naidoo and Wills, 2016). It had a behaviourist approach (stimulus and response) as it was anticipated that knowledge equated to behaviour change (Niven, 2006). It was neither holistic nor a person-centred approach; the social determinants of health were ignored and the emphasis placed on individual responsibility rather than any external influences, such as governmental or societal influences (Scriven, 2017).

Scriven (2017) suggests that health education today is a planned opportunity; for example, the DAFNE programme (Dose Adjustment For Normal Eating) for people with type 1 diabetes or the Moving Forward course after treatment for breast cancer. It is now an approach where the health promoter is a facilitator and emphasis is placed on collaborative and partnership working between the health promoter and the individual/community, where empowerment and informed choices are key (Naidoo and Wills, 2016).

6.11.2 Empowerment

The NHS Long Term Plan (2019) places emphasis on empowerment, not only of clinical staff but also of our service users/patients. As a nursing associate, you are expected to empower individuals, families and communities so that they can make informed choices to change their health behaviours, which contributes to improving their health and reducing or eradicating health inequalities (NMC, 2018a; NMC, 2018b).

Empowerment is defined by Naidoo and Wills (2016, p. 75) as *"the act of acquiring power and the ability to make decisions and take control over one's life"*. Empowering others will require you to use a range of person-centred health promotion theories and models. This may also include signposting them to appropriate services, practical activities and potentially supporting them to increase their self-confidence and self-worth (self-esteem), encourage the belief that they can change their health behaviours and have the resources to do so (self-efficacy) and that they can take control of their lives which relates to their own internal locus of control (see *Section 5.9*) (Knight, 2020).

6.11.3 Healthy and empowering conversations

Making Every Contact Count (MECC) is an opportunistic approach that can also be used for planned health promotion interventions, which uses Healthy Conversation Skills. MECC is:

> *"... an approach to behaviour change that uses the millions of day-to-day interactions that organisations and people have with other people to support them in making positive changes to their physical and mental health and wellbeing. MECC enables the opportunistic delivery of consistent and concise healthy lifestyle information and enables individuals to engage in conversations about their health at scale across organisations and populations" (PHE et al., 2016, p. 6).*

It is a brief evidence-based intervention that can take place within a few seconds to two minutes (a very brief intervention) or from two to five minutes (a brief intervention) (PHE *et al.*, 2016). It is a person-centred approach in which you facilitate a discussion with people where they can identify for themselves what health and wellbeing issues are important to them. It values their unique experience and self-knowledge and uses both healthy conversation skills and shared decision-making. Supporting individuals to develop their self-efficacy is embedded within MECC and, even if people choose not to change their behaviour as a result of the intervention, they are more in control of their health and understanding of it, which empowers them.

The four principles that support healthy conversation skills (Mecc-z-card, 2020) are:

- People are responsible for their own choices.
- Being given information alone does not make people change.
- People come to us with solutions (although they may be unable to enact these solutions due to difficulties accessing services such as healthcare or housing, or a lack of financial support to improve diet and nutrition).
- It is not possible to persuade people to change their habit.

ACTIVITY 6.6

Reflect on these four behavioural principles and then consider how you feel about them.

The key to using MECC is effective communication (see *Section 2.2*), and importance is placed on what the person wants to achieve for their health and wellbeing and not what the health professional thinks they should achieve. This can be a challenge for health professionals as they can sometimes feel that, as the 'expert', they know what is best for an individual (Knight, 2020).

MECC provides guidance on the response styles that you need to hold a Healthy Conversation. These include the use of open questions, especially beginning questions with How and What, also known as Open Discovery Questions (ODQs) (Lawrence, 2021). The use of these is essential so that relevant information can be obtained. If you use a closed question such as "Do you like vegetables?" the answer can be only yes or no, whereas asking "What vegetables do you like?" will enable the individual to specify their vegetable likes and dislikes. Sometimes a closed question is useful; for example, "Do you have access to a cooker?"

Other important skills are those of empathy and reflection (Mecc-z-card, 2020). Empathy means that you demonstrate that you understand the individual and/or the family situation they are going through, using your emotional intelligence (Edwards, 2001; Walsh, 2018). Empathy can be displayed by non-verbal body language and active listening. It can also be strengthened by considering the wider factors which influence their individual health behaviours. Reflection can be considered in two ways during a healthy conversation. One aspect is reflecting back to the person what you understand them to have said, which clarifies not only your understanding but also theirs; this also demonstrates active listening. The other aspect is to reflect on the conversation itself. This can be during the conversation, so you can change your approach as needed (reflection-in-action) and also by taking time afterwards to reflect on the interaction and what you did well and what you would do differently next time (reflection-on-action) (Schön, 1982).

» **In addition to communication skills, empathy and reflection are important to Making Every Contact Count.**

It may be appropriate sometimes to say "In my experience…"; for example, "In my experience, as a nursing associate, I have seen that attending the cardiac rehabilitation clinic has given patients confidence to resume exercise and other activities". In addition, telling and suggesting can have a part to play; for example, if someone has identified they want to give up smoking you can signpost them to the local smoking cessation services (Mecc-z-card, 2020).

An important part of MECC is to support the individual to set a goal using the SMARTER framework (Specific, Measurable, Achievable, Relevant, Time-bound, Evaluated and Reviewed).

CASE STUDY 6.1 USING ODQS AND SMARTER

Clara is 25 years old and works as a secretary for a legal firm. She has been living on her own for the first time in a rented one-bedroom flat in an area that she moved to three months ago. She now lives 150 miles away from her family. Clara has told you at an appointment for an assessment relating to her asthma that she is very lonely and is also aware that her alcohol consumption has increased significantly since moving. She drinks every night after work as it is easy to buy alcohol on the way home from work as she walks past an off-licence. She also smokes 10–20 cigarettes a day.

- What ODQs could you ask Clara?
- Which goal do you think Clara might decide to choose?

Using the SMARTER model how could she plan to meet this goal? Remember it needs to be Specific, Measurable, Achievable, Relevant, Time-bound, Evaluated and Reviewed (HEE, 2017).

In summary, for you to use MECC to hold a healthy conversation you need to:
1. "Use Open Discovery Questions to help someone explore an issue.
2. Reflect on your practice and conversations.
3. Spend more time listening than giving information or making suggestions.
4. Use Open Discovery Questions to support someone to make a SMARTER plan." (Mecc-z-card, 2020).

This section only provides an overview of MECC. To use it effectively you need to undertake a recognised Royal Society of Public Health accredited course.

6.12 Understanding some of the challenges to changing health behaviour

There are many challenges that individuals feel they face when trying to change their health behaviours, which may include access to resources, possibly associated with the social determinants of health; for example, lack of money to join a gym or poor access to transport to shop for food in a supermarket or market, rather than locally which can be more expensive. These aspects need to be considered when using the healthy conversation skills and setting SMARTER goals. Other challenges relate to individual beliefs and attitudes and that is why it is helpful to understand the health belief model and the theory of reasoned action.

6.12.1 Health Belief Model

The decision whether to make a health behaviour change, or not, is based on the individual's perception of their:

- Perceived susceptibility (Am I vulnerable?)
- Perceived severity (Am I at risk or in danger?)
- Perceived benefits (What is in it for me? What are the advantages?)
- Perceived barriers (What are the disadvantages and what are my obstacles?)
- Cue to action (What is prompting me to act?)
- Self-efficacy.

(Knight, 2020, p. 125; adapted from: Strecher and Rosenstock, 1997, pp. 113–114)

ACTIVITY 6.7

Refer back to *Case study 6.1*.

It is important as a health promoter that if Clara was considering reducing her alcohol intake you understand what her beliefs are. What do you think her beliefs might be, linked to each aspect of the Health Belief Model?

Perceived susceptibility: e.g. risk of liver disease

Perceived severity:

Perceived benefits:

Perceived barriers:

Cue to action:

Her self-efficacy:

6.12.2 Theory of Reasoned Action

Ajzen and Fishbein's (1980) Theory of Reasoned Action recognises that the behaviour of an individual is influenced by their attitude. Scott (2020, p. 46) explains that this "... *theory assumes that people use rational decision-making to underpin reasoned action*". The concept of perceived 'social norms' is relevant as well. Think about Clara who acknowledges that she is drinking too much; implicit in this is her understanding that this is not beneficial for her health. Her perception may be based on influences from her friends (although Clara has identified she is lonely), her family, her community (both at home and in the workplace), her level of education and her culture. What her perceived 'norms' are will influence whether she wants to, and will, reduce her alcohol intake. You as the health promoter can find out what her attitude is using ODQs.

ACTIVITY 6.8

What ODQ(s) could you ask Clara to find out her attitudes and beliefs about alcohol?

6.12.3 The Transtheoretical Model or Stages of Change Model

The Transtheoretical Model or Stages of Change Model, formulated by Prochaska and DiClemente (1986), presents change as a five-stage process; precontemplation, contemplation, preparing to change, making the change and maintaining the change. Let us explore how this model can be applied to Clara in *Table 6.1*.

Table 6.1 *The Transtheoretical / Stages of Change Model; adapted from Prochaska and DiClemente (1986)*

Stage of Change	Clara
Precontemplation	At this stage Clara would not be considering that she needs to change her health behaviours, e.g. related to alcohol consumption or smoking.
Contemplation	From the case study, we know that Clara is at this stage as she is aware that her alcohol consumption has increased significantly since moving.
Preparing to change	Here Clara has set her SMARTER goal to reduce her alcohol consumption by only drinking alcohol at the weekend and is planning how she will achieve this (e.g. changing the route home from work so she does not pass the off-licence, joining a gym and going there straight from work, or joining a club or organisation where she can meet and make friends). Signposting might be needed here by the health promoter, e.g. to local gyms or clubs as Clara is new to the area.

Table 6.1 (continued)

Stage of Change	Clara
Making the change	Clara has implemented her chosen actions to achieve her goal.
Maintenance	Clara has achieved her goal of reducing her alcohol intake and now only drinks socially when she is out with her new friends at weekends. For it to be considered a sustained health behaviour change it needs to be continued for 6 months or more.

Although the table suggests that the Transtheoretical model is linear, it is not. Individuals may relapse back and then move forwards again (e.g. Clara might start drinking every day again) and as a health promoter you need to be aware that an individual has the freedom to choose. However, this does not mean that Clara, or anyone, will not achieve a permanent change sometime in the future.

ACTIVITY 6.9

Refer back to *Activity 6.1*. Having read this chapter, choose one outcome from the NMC (2018a) *Standards of Proficiency for Nursing Associates* that you do not feel confident in and make an action plan to achieve it. Standards are available at: www.nmc.org.uk/standards/standards-for-nursing-associates/standards-of-proficiency-for-nursing-associates or bit.ly/3Z8XZ6V

CHAPTER SUMMARY

- Knowledge and understanding of public health and health promotion theories are essential to your role as a nursing associate.
- Public health and health promotion are essential for improving health outcomes, reducing health inequalities and health protection.
- Empowering others will require you to use a range of person-centred health promotion theories and models.
- Every day you have the opportunity to hold healthy conversations, using MECC, with the people you come into contact with, to help them improve their health.

FURTHER READING

Bennett, C. and Lillyman, S. (eds) (2020) *Promoting Health and Wellbeing: for nursing and healthcare students.* Lantern Publishing.

Knight, A., La Placa, V. and McNaught, A. (eds) (2014) *Wellbeing: policy and practice.* Lantern Publishing.

Naidoo, J. and Wills, J. (2016) *Foundations for Health Promotion*, 4th edition. Elsevier.

Scriven, A. (2017) *Ewles & Simnett's Promoting Health: a practical guide*, 7th edition. Elsevier.

References

Acheson, D. (1988) *Public Health in England: report to the committee of inquiry into the future of the public health function.* HMSO.

Ajzen, I. and Fishbein, M. (1980) *Understanding Attitudes and Predicting Social Behavior.* Prentice-Hall.

Edwards, S.D. (2001) *Philosophy of Nursing: an introduction.* Palgrave.

Gov.UK (2020) *Government creates new National Institute for Health Protection.* Press release. Available at: www.gov.uk/government/news/government-creates-new-national-institute-for-health-protection (accessed 7 December 2022).

Gov.UK (2021) UK Health Security Agency. Available at: www.gov.uk/government/organisations/uk-health-security-agency (accessed 7 December 2022).

HEE (2017) *Health Education England Wessex Making Every Contact Count Healthy Conversation Skills Training Manual.* Health Education England.

Knight, A. (2020) 'Building a Healthy Public Policy'. In Bennett, C. and Lillyman, S. (eds) (2020) *Promoting Health and Wellbeing: for nursing and healthcare students.* Lantern Publishing.

Lawrence, W. (2021) Teaching practitioners Healthy Conversation Skills. Available at: https://practicalhealthpsychology.com/2021/03/how-to-support-patients-to-lose-weight-and-better-manage-their-type-2-diabetes or bit.ly/3y2bgSR (accessed 5 January 2023).

Mecc-z-card (2020) Available at: www.healthyconversationskills.co.uk/uploads/mecc-z-card-dec20-final.pdf or bit.ly/3UJGby8 (accessed 17 April 2023).

Naidoo, J. and Wills, J. (2016) *Foundations for Health Promotion*, 4th edition. Elsevier.

NHS (2019) *The NHS Long Term Plan.* Available at: www.longtermplan.nhs.uk/publication/nhs-long-term-plan (accessed 7 December 2022).

NHS England (2014) *Five Year Forward View.* Available at: www.england.nhs.uk/wp-content/uploads/2014/10/5yfv-web.pdf or bit.ly/3U7261C (accessed 7 December 2022).

NHS England (2017) *Next Steps on the NHS Five Year Forward View.* Available at: www.england.nhs.uk/wp-content/uploads/2017/03/NEXT-STEPS-ON-THE-NHS-FIVE-YEAR-FORWARD-VIEW.pdf or bit.ly/3ENiK05 (accessed 7 December 2022).

NICE (2019) *Glossary.* National Institute for Health and Care Excellence. Available at: www.nice.org.uk/Glossary?letter=H (accessed 7 December 2022).

Niven, N. (2006) *The Psychology of Nursing Care.* Palgrave Macmillan.

NMC (2018a) *Standards of Proficiency for Nursing Associates.* Nursing and Midwifery Council.

NMC (2018b) *The Code: professional standards of practice and behaviour for nurses, midwives and nursing associates.* Nursing and Midwifery Council.

Parliament UK (2020) *Living Heritage. People and Parliament Transforming Society. 1942 Beveridge Report.* Available at: www.parliament.uk/about/living-heritage/transformingsociety/livinglearning/coll-9-health1/coll-9-health or bit.ly/3mapiiF (accessed 7 December 2022).

Prochaska, J.O. and DiClemente, C.C. (1986) 'Toward a comprehensive model of change'. In Miller, W.R. and Heather, N. (eds) *Treating Addictive Behaviors: processes of change*. Plenum Press.

Public Health England [PHE] (2020) *About us*. Available at: www.gov.uk/government/organisations/public-health-england/about (accessed 7 December 2022).

Public Health England [PHE], NHS England and Health Education England (2016) *Making Every Contact Count (MECC): Consensus statement*. Available at: www.england.nhs.uk/wp-content/uploads/2016/04/making-every-contact-count.pdf (accessed 7 December 2022).

Schön, D. (1982) *The Reflective Practitioner: how professionals think in action*. Routledge.

Scott, S. (2020) 'Behaviour change: theories, models and approaches'. In Bennett, C. and Lillyman, S. (eds) *Promoting Health and Wellbeing: for nursing and healthcare students*. Lantern Publishing.

Scriven, A. (2017) *Ewles & Simnett's Promoting Health: a practical guide*, 7th edition. Elsevier.

Steel, N., Ford, J., Newton, J. *et al.* (2018) Changes in health in the countries of the UK and 150 English Local Authority areas 1990–2016: a systematic analysis for the Global Burden of Disease Study 2016. *The Lancet*, **392** (10158): 1647–1661.

Strecher, V.J. and Rosenstock, I.M. (1997) 'The health belief model'. In Baum, A., Newman, S., Weinman, J. *et al.* (eds) *Cambridge Handbook of Psychology, Health and Medicine*. Cambridge University Press.

Walsh, M. (2018) *Key Topics in Social Sciences: an A–Z guide for student nurses*. Lantern Publishing.

Wanless, D. (2004) *Securing Good Health for the Whole Population: final report*. Department of Health.

WHO (1978) *Declaration of Alma-Ata*. Available at: https://cdn.who.int/media/docs/default-source/documents/almaata-declaration-en.pdf?sfvrsn=7b3c2167_2 or bit.ly/3F9ga4L (accessed 9 January 2023).

WHO (1986) *The Ottawa Charter for Health Promotion*. World Health Organization. Available at: www.who.int/publications/i/item/ottawa-charter-for-health-promotion or bit.ly/3m4M4c6 (accessed 7 December 2022).

WHO (1998) *Health Literacy*. Available at: www.who.int/activities/improving-health-literacy (accessed 7 December 2022).

WHO (2006) *Health Promotion*. World Health Organization. Available at: www.who.int/topics/health_promotion/en (accessed 7 December 2022).

WHO (2009) *Milestones in Health Promotion: statements from global conferences*. World Health Organization. Available at: www.who.int/publications/i/item/WHO-NMH-CHP-09.01 (accessed 7 December 2022).

WHO (2020) *What we do*. World Health Organization. Available at: www.who.int/about/what-we-do (accessed 7 December 2022).

WHO Regional Office for Europe (2020) *Public Health Services*. Available at: www.euro.who.int/en/health-topics/Health-systems/public-health-services/public-health-services or bit.ly/3KRkQjn (accessed 7 December 2022).

7

RESEARCH AND EVIDENCE-BASED PRACTICE

Neil Davison and David Matthews

This chapter relates to outcome 1.7 within the
Standards of Proficiency for Nursing Associates **(NMC, 2018).**

LEARNING OUTCOMES

When you have completed this chapter you should be able to:
- Define the terms 'research' and 'evidence-based practice'.
- Outline the research process.
- Describe the key features of research methodologies and define validity and reliability.
- Appreciate the role of critical appraisal when reading research reports.
- Outline how research studies fit within the hierarchy of evidence used to inform evidence-based practice.
- Describe how evidence-based practice supports the role of the nursing associate.

7.1 Introduction

This chapter introduces research and evidence-based practice and will help you to "describe the principles of research and how research findings are used to inform evidence-based practice", as required by the standards of proficiency for nursing associates (NMC, 2018, p. 5). Initially sources of nursing knowledge are discussed and the research process outlined. The chapter then introduces the various research methods, supported by examples from clinical practice. The relationship between research and evidence-based practice is explored and the role that critical appraisal plays in enhancing knowledge for practice is discussed.

7.2 The knowledge base of nursing practice

Nursing practice is based on knowledge drawn from many subject areas, e.g. anatomy and physiology, psychology, microbiology and pharmacology.

Knowledge is also derived from research studies about nursing. Some historical sources of knowledge are less obvious but may still influence practice.

- Tradition: We've always done it this way
- Sister says: Nurses were instructed by a senior member of staff
- Expert opinion: From books, articles, tuition or demonstration
- Trial and error: Various methods were attempted until one worked well.

The latter third of the twentieth century saw a demand for a more robust source of knowledge to improve the quality and effectiveness of care provided to patients. Research offered a method of achieving this and it became more prevalent in nursing practice and education. Research is "any enquiry that is systematic in its approach and that seeks to ensure that the results of the enquiry cannot be criticised on the grounds of poor techniques" (Jolley, 2020, p. 4). The systematic part of the enquiry is the 'research process' outlined below. Research aims to allow nursing to build a body of knowledge (Grove, Gray and Burns, 2015). Nurses were increasingly educated to be research-minded and aware, but applying research-generated knowledge to nursing practice remained a challenge. Towards the end of the twentieth century evidence-based practice (EBP) emerged as not only a means of providing nurses and other healthcare professionals with evidence on which to base their practice, but also a process that examined the quality of the research.

7.3 The research process

The research process has three key parts each containing a series of activities:

- Identifying the research question
- Collecting the data
- Analysing the data and disseminating results.

7.3.1 Identifying the research question

The research question: This might arise from an observation or question of everyday clinical practice, from the need to develop evidence-based practice or in response to a call from a funding body such as The King's Fund or the National Institute for Health Research.

Searching and evaluating the literature: This stage identifies what is already known about the question, as it may have already been answered by a previous study.

Choosing a methodology and research design: This depends on the research question. If the research was trying to establish which wound dressing used for leg ulcers was considered most comfortable by sufferers, then a survey may be appropriate. If the study looked to explore what life is like with a leg ulcer, then one of the qualitative approaches would be suitable.

Preparing a research proposal: This is a statement of what the research intends to do, when it will be done and how often. It will also detail the costs of the study for the funding body or could be used to secure a grant for the research.

7.3.2 Collecting the data

Accessing the data: Conducting research in healthcare involves access to sensitive data, vulnerable individuals and requires confidentiality. To ensure that proposed research meets the standards necessary in the UK, all proposals are scrutinised by panels of experts for ethical, legal and scientific rigour.

Sampling: This stage of the process involves choosing the sample and its size. Generally, quantitative research methods use larger samples than qualitative.

Pilot study: This is a small-scale version of the study using a sample similar to that which will be used for the main study. It is designed to iron out any problems and to make sure that the tools used to gather data perform as expected. The tools could be an interview schedule, a questionnaire used in a survey or a scale that measures pain.

Collecting data: This stage of the process is where observations of behaviour, questionnaire completion or in-depth interviews take place, depending on the research methodology.

7.3.3 Analysing the data, disseminating results and implementing findings

Analysing the data: Numerical data is subjected to statistical analysis and text from interviews is analysed for patterns and themes.

Disseminating results: Results from the research need to be shared with fellow professionals, patients and service providers. Traditionally this has been done through conferences, publication in academic journals and seminars, but publication on university websites, patient information group websites as well as social media channels allows access to a wider audience.

Implementing findings: Healthcare-related research studies usually include a statement on the implications of the results for practice, education and research. This helps to guide nurses on the implementation of findings. Organisations such as the National Institute for Health and Care Excellence (NICE) also

» NICE is an organisation that seeks to improve the quality of care and health outcomes for users of the NHS and health and social care services.

support healthcare professionals in the implementation of research findings by evaluating research studies and developing evidence-based practice. NICE (www.nice.org.uk) produces evidence-based guidance for health professionals and the wider public. It aims to ensure that users have access to quality health and social care services, irrespective of where they live in the UK, and that those services provided are based on the best evidence and represent value for money.

ACTIVITY 7.1

Select a journal that you have read to keep up to date or to gain information for an assignment, and check the list of contents to find a research report. Use this outline of the research process to help navigate through the report.

RECAP

- Research offers a method of achieving a robust source of knowledge to improve the quality and effectiveness of care provided to patients.
- The research process has three key parts:
  1. Identifying the research question
  2. Collecting the data
  3. Analysing the data and disseminating results.

7.4 Evidence-based practice

Evidence-based practice can be viewed as "the integration of the best possible research evidence with clinical expertise and with patient needs" (Porter-O'Grady, 2006, p. 1).

The EBP approach has the advantage over research alone in that:
- It is patient-focused.
- It values clinical decision-making.
- It recognises that a single research study may be unable to address many issues arising in nursing practice.
- It acknowledges that some perspectives of patients' experiences may not be researchable via clinical trials.

(Schmidt and Brown, 2019)

7.5 Research

Understanding the fundamentals of research is a prerequisite to appreciating the role of EBP in nursing. Nursing involves applying knowledge and technical skills in a compassionate and sensitive manner to a patient, a unique and individual human being. This relationship and process is complex but if viewed in a simplified way, two broad areas can be seen. First there are the skills, treatment and products used, for example, when caring for a wound. Do they speed up the healing process; do they reduce discomfort; are they cost-effective? Secondly, there is the experience of the patient within the care process. What is it like to have a chronic wound; how does it affect daily life; does it prevent sufferers from socialising? Different research methods are needed to increase the knowledge base of our practice.

7.5.1 Quantitative research

Quantitative research is a systematic process that describes variables and the relationship between them or identifies cause and effect between variables (Grove, Gray and Burns, 2015).

Variables

Independent variable

The independent variable is manipulated or changed in the research study. If a study sought to find out if patients listening to music reported less pain than those who didn't, the playing of music is the independent variable.

Dependent variable

This is changed by the independent variable. In the example above, the dependent variable is the amount of pain reported by patients.

Extraneous variables

These are all variables other than the independent and dependent ones that could influence the result of the research study. In the ideal circumstances, these would be controlled so they did not interfere with the results, as in an experiment. If a research study was examining whether certain treatment and wound care products used accelerated the healing process and reduced discomfort in a chronic wound, then the extraneous variables might include different anxiety levels between patients, different reasons for their pain, the surroundings where they are being treated and even the room temperature and décor.

Wong *et al.* (2020) explored the effect of transcutaneous electrical nerve stimulation (TENS) on pain during dressing changes performed on leg ulcers in 28 patients with painful and complicated wounds. Pain intensity was measured numerically before the procedure and at the point during the procedure when patients requested the TENS to be switched on. The sample used was quite small but it found that TENS did reduce the intensity of pain experienced.

Population

A population is the total number of individuals from which data could be collected. In most research studies it is not practical to gather data from the entire population. A population could be every registered nursing associate, every pre-operative patient or everyone with a venous leg ulcer. The exception to this is the population census, taken every 10 years, where the entire population of England and Wales is asked questions and required to supply data.

Quantitative research methods usually aim to find answers in an objective and impartial way by testing a hypothesis. The hypothesis is a statement about the expected relationship between variables; for example, the use of a wound dressing that creates a moist wound environment will reduce the time taken for the wound to heal.

Sample

This is a carefully selected portion of the population representative of the characteristics of the population, such as age and gender.

Hypothesis

This is a statement about the relationship between two or more variables, such as music and pain in the earlier example. The hypothesis may be stated as:

'Patients who listen to music will experience less pain intensity than those who do not'.

Data produced is in a numerical form and the hypothesis is accepted or rejected based on statistical analysis. If the sample used in the research is truly representative of the population, then the results can be generalised back to the population.

Data

Data comprises facts or information collected during a research study for the purpose of analysis. In quantitative research data is usually numerical; in qualitative research data is usually in the form of text.

Experiments

Experiments are conducted in a controlled environment where one or more independent variables are manipulated and the effect on the dependent variable observed and measured. As well as an experimental group who receive the treatment there is a control group who do not, or who receive a placebo treatment instead. The study subjects are assigned to the experimental or control group randomly.

Sometimes it is impossible to carry out true experiments in the clinical environment. This may be because randomisation of the study or control group is not possible, or for ethical reasons. If an experiment cannot meet all of the features of a true experiment such as control and randomisation, it is referred to as quasi-experimental.

Ylonen *et al.* (2017) researched the effectiveness of an internet-based educational programme about venous leg ulcers using a quasi-experimental design. The study found that e-learning programmes do increase nurses' knowledge but only in the short term, indicating a need for continuous education.

Randomised controlled trials

Randomised controlled trials (RCTs) are viewed as providing high quality of evidence for EBP. These are experiments where participants are randomly assigned to the experimental or control group and form the basis of clinical trials. Guest *et al.* (2018) investigated the cost-effectiveness of a device placed close to non-healing venous leg ulcers. The device discharged a micro electrical current and the effect of this on the healing rate was studied using a randomised controlled trial. The experimental group of 43 used functioning devices whereas the control group of 47 used identical placebo devices. While some patients reported improvements with the micro current device, the trial did not demonstrate the cost-effectiveness of it.

Meta-analysis

This method involves the re-analysis of data from a number of combined studies and offers the highest quality of evidence for EBP. Studies used in the re-analysis must meet specific inclusion criteria. Minyan Zhao *et al.* (2020) performed a meta-analysis of eight randomised controlled trials involving 1057 participants, investigating the use of silver dressings for healing venous leg ulcers. The meta-analysis showed that in the short term, there is evidence that silver dressings speed up the healing of chronic venous leg ulcers. However, it recommended that more studies are needed to explore the effect of silver dressings on total wound healing in the longer term.

Surveys

A survey collects data by obtaining responses to questions from a sample of individuals. A survey may be self-completed, as with a questionnaire, or questions are read out and responses recorded by an interviewer. Quantitative data may be obtained using numerically rated items or scales, but open-ended questions can be used to yield qualitative data. Lindsay (2018) used a patient satisfaction survey to ascertain the experiences and views of members, the leg club name for patients attending a leg ulcer clinic. Members rated aspects of the care and service offered by the leg club, providing numerical data for analysis. They were also asked open-ended questions such as 'what is it like living with a leg ulcer?', yielding varied responses such as pain, discomfort and being physically restricted.

Leren *et al.* (2021) used a questionnaire as part of a study that explored the proportion of people with leg ulcers who suffer with pain from their ulcer in everyday life. The study found that 64% of those who took part in the study experienced pain, and this was linked with older age, being female and having a reduced quality of sleep. The study highlighted the need for pain assessment and management in people with leg ulcers.

7.5.2 Qualitative research

Qualitative research uses a systematic approach to describe life experiences. It aims to gain understanding and meaning from the situations and interactions that involve individuals and to develop theories that describe and explain these. This approach to research believes that individuals interact with and within their natural environment, and their experiences need to be studied within this. Qualitative research generates data that is not usually quantifiable in numbers.

Phenomenology

Phenomenology is a method in qualitative research that is suited to exploring a patient's experience of illness and care. Interviews are used to elicit how the respondent makes sense of their experience, and respondents are able to talk freely. Questions are asked to clarify or explore issues raised by the respondent but answers are not limited, as in a survey. Data is analysed by looking for trends and themes within the respondent's narrative replies and presented using direct quotes to support the themes. Hopkins (2004) explored the experiences and coping strategies of five people living with non-healing leg ulcers. They were asked to complete a diary and had an unstructured interview based on the question: 'What is it like to live with non-healing venous leg ulcers?' The participants had lived with leg ulcers for between 3 and 45 years. Results indicated that the effect of living with long-term venous leg ulcers should not be viewed as only a physical problem.

Lernevall *et al.* (2017) investigated the everyday experiences of patients with arterial or mixed leg ulcers by interviewing six patients. Respondents described being in a living hell, with death preferable to spending the remainder of their lives with a leg ulcer. The results suggested that the person with the wound needed treatment, not just the wound.

Grounded theory

This qualitative approach generates theory during the study, which may then be explored further within the same study. It is characterised by the simultaneous collection and analysis of data and is usually used to explain social relationships and behaviours.

For example, a study may seek to explore the experience of people with painful leg ulcers using in-depth interviews. The leg ulcer sufferers talk about administrative problems at their GP practices in getting regular prescriptions for strong pain relief, so the next phase of the study focuses on interviewing GPs and practice managers.

Lagerin, Hylander and Törnkvist (2017) used grounded theory to investigate the experiences of district nurses in Sweden caring for patients with leg ulcers in accordance with clinical guidelines. This was achieved by conducting semi-structured group interviews with 30 nurses. The results showed that nurses try to work within the guidelines but experience obstacles, particularly when trying to keep patients motivated when little healing progress was being made. Overcoming patients' feelings of hopelessness also challenged their adherence to clinical guidelines.

Ethnography

Ethnography aims to describe people, their habits, customs and cultures from their point of view. The study of people in their own environment is achieved by participant observation and face-to-face interviews. Lauzon Clabo (2007) used an ethnographic approach when studying how nurses on two surgical wards assessed pain. This involved collecting data over nine months using several methods including participant observation. The researcher worked alongside the study subjects over a period of time while gathering data. This was to try to minimise the effect of being observed as the researcher has become part of the daily routine.

ACTIVITY 7.2

A new male urology day unit is planned to replace the rather old and cramped one in your local hospital. It is due to open in 12 months and has to meet the needs of its many older, catheterised patients. Take a few minutes to consider which research method might be most appropriate to find out what services, support and advice users see as essential.

A questionnaire given out to patients visiting the current unit may provide some useful information, but patients may be preoccupied or anxious about their treatment and not concentrate on the questionnaire or complete it. The questionnaire may seek responses about what the researcher considers to be important services, support and advice as they have designed the questionnaire. The views of the researcher may be substantially different from those of patients.

Alternatively, a sample of the patients could be invited to a focus group where more detailed, in-depth responses can be obtained. These could be used as a basis for a questionnaire to a larger sample of patients who would be asked to agree/disagree or rank the usefulness of proposed services, support and advice.

ACTIVITY 7.3

From their considerable experience of caring for patients with venous leg ulcers, the district nursing team noticed that those patients who manage to elevate their ulcerated leg for long periods of time throughout the day seem to have faster-healing ulcers than patients who elevate for shorter periods. Consider which research method might be used to investigate the observation made by the district nursing team.

The variables involved in this investigation, the rate of ulcer healing and leg elevation are measurable. This problem could be investigated using a quasi-experimental design. The experimental group of patients elevate their ulcerated legs for a specified minimum amount of time daily and the rate of healing is measured. The control group would contain patients who elevate their ulcerated legs for their usual amount of time but below the specified minimum time. What this doesn't tell us is why some patients are unable to elevate their ulcerated leg. Patients may have other responsibilities such as caring for an ailing partner which may lead to self-neglect.

Occasionally a research study will use quantitative and qualitative methods. Probst *et al.* (2020) studied the experiences of people with venous leg ulcers and their understanding of why the ulcer may reoccur after healing. They combined quantitative and qualitative methods of data collection in the form of questionnaires and interviews. This is referred to as a mixed methods approach. The study found that in 145 participants, venous leg ulcers recurred in 33% of them over a 12-month period, frequently following accidental skin damage.

7.5.3 Critical appraisal

Critical appraisal is about assessing whether the results of research are able to inform practice. Critical appraisal helps to develop and improve the knowledge base of nursing by weeding out practices that are wasteful of time and resources or may be harmful. It is important to be balanced in the judgement of practices, and new methods or innovations should be subjected to the same level of scrutiny as more historic parts of nursing practice. Rees, Beecroft and Booth (2015) suggest that good research studies provide sufficient information for the reader to assess that the study is good, but caution that poor quality studies may not carry a warning. This means that you have to make judgements about what you read. Some help is available from one of the many critical appraisal tools or checklists designed to help evaluate research evidence. Some checklists are intended for non-research-based evidence and many are specialised to one type of study, for example a qualitative study or meta-analysis. A link to critical appraisal tools is given in the further reading section at the end of the chapter.

As a starting point, considering the following points and questions when reading a research study will help you to develop critical appraisal skills.

>> **Critical appraisal involves making judgements about what you read in order to assess whether the results of research can inform practice.**

Where was the study published?

Academic journals publish research studies and subject them to review by peers before publication. This doesn't automatically mean that all published papers are perfect. You may find reports of research studies on university websites, news websites, social media channels and even household magazines, but these will not provide sufficient detail for you to evaluate them.

Who are the authors?

At the beginning of the paper there are details about the author(s), their qualifications, positions, employment and area of expertise.

The title of the study

Does it communicate what the research is about?

What is the purpose of the paper?

Is it easy to grasp what the research question is? If there is a hypothesis, is it written clearly? Are the aims and objectives of the study stated? Can you understand what the researcher is going to investigate and how?

The literature review

This section discusses published evidence of what is known about the subject of the study. It will also identify areas where knowledge is lacking and make links to the purpose and need for the current study as well as the method of investigation. The literature review should be comprehensive and reflect current knowledge, so expect to see literature that has been published very recently. Don't be alarmed by seeing some older publication dates, as there will be classic studies or key papers that inform the knowledge base of all subjects. Ideally the original published literature should have been read as part of the review. Secondary references, where a researcher's work is cited in another publication, have the risk of being influenced by another author's judgement or may miss out key details.

The research methodology

The investigation will be designed around one of the research methods outlined earlier in this chapter. It is worth considering whether the chosen approach seems the most appropriate way of finding out about the subject. The variables under investigation, for example pain or urinary incontinence, will be defined and how they will be measured explained. Frequently researched variables such as urinary incontinence have a standardised international definition, so check to see if there is one for the variable that you are reading about. The research method and any data collection tools need to be valid and reliable.

Validity

Validity refers to the extent to which the research actually measures what it intends to measure. A study could measure the amount of pain that patients experienced by asking them to rate their pain on a pain scale, where 0 equals no pain and 10 equals the worst pain imaginable. Alternatively, the amount of pain experienced by patients could be measured by looking at medication charts to find out how much pain relief they were given. The first study asks patients to decide how much pain they have, so it is seen as having validity. The second study could be measuring the availability of nurses to administer pain relief, the nature of the nurse–patient relationship, the opinions and attitudes of nurses towards pain relief or that patients may want to be seen as brave and not weak, and therefore lacks validity.

Reliability

If a research method or scale is reliable, it achieves similar results each time it is used. This can be considered as consistency in measurement; a scale measuring patient's pain is expected to be reliable, as are bathroom scales.

Does the sample represent the population?

Reading the section on sampling should explain how the sample used for the study was arrived at and to what extent any results are generalisable back to the population that it represents. Remember that qualitative research methods use smaller samples than quantitative ones.

What ethical considerations were made?

Healthcare research frequently involves staff or patients and possibly their families. Research proposals are subjected to scrutiny by an ethics committee to ensure that the rights of individuals are protected whether they choose or refuse to take part in a study. Researchers and members of ethics committees are guided and informed by national guidelines. Researchers will also be expected to store and manage patient data in a confidential and secure manner.

Data collection

Details of the method of gathering data will be provided, allowing you to consider potential strengths and weaknesses. For example, observing participants may influence their behaviour; a researcher has no control over who actually completes a questionnaire, whereas interviewing participants allows for follow-up questions to clarify responses and increases the detail in respondents' answers.

Results

Numerical results are reported as figures, averages and percentages within the text of the report as well as in table and diagrammatic form. Results from qualitative studies include extracts of text from interview questions, focus group discussions or diary entries. Are the results of the study clearly presented?

Implications of the results

The researcher may make recommendations based on the findings of their study. Do any suggested actions, such as a change in practice or further research, seem reasonable based on the results you have read?

Conclusions

The conclusion should draw together discussions about the findings of the research study. The researcher may highlight weaknesses in the study that need to be considered alongside the results, so read carefully.

References

Research studies usually have a comprehensive reference list to other related literature and research. This can be a useful source of reading material if you are studying the same subject.

7.6 The hierarchy of evidence

EBP is intended to offer high quality, cost-effective care for patients. Therefore the information used to inform the evidence base needs to be of a high standard. This leads to the development of a hierarchy, often displayed as a pyramid with the highest quality evidence at the apex and the lowest quality at the base (*Figure 7.1*). Evidence within the hierarchy includes expert opinion and the various methods of research.

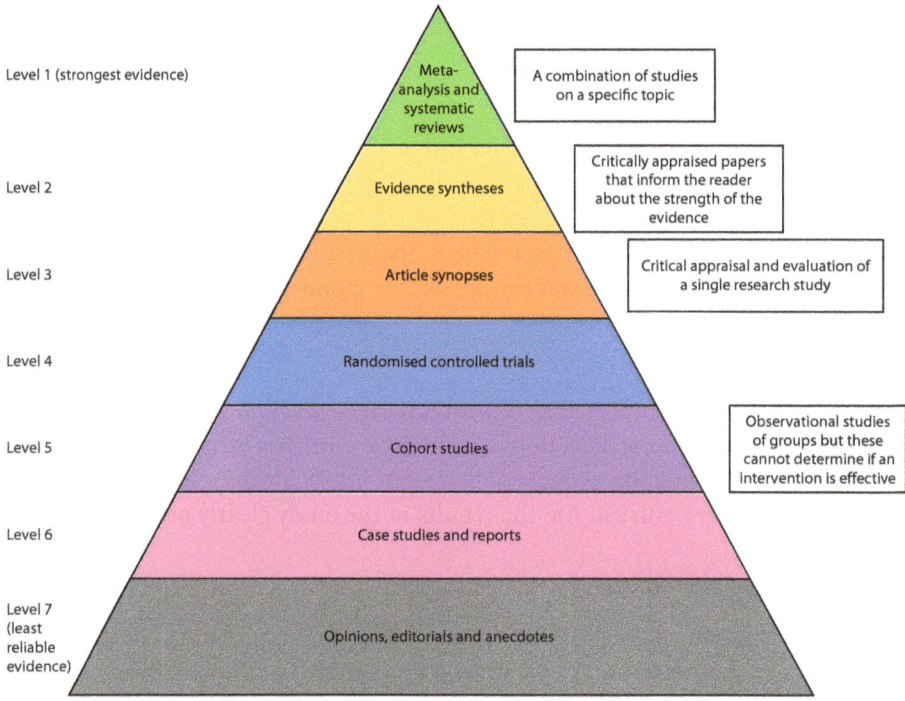

Level 1 (strongest evidence) — Meta-analysis and systematic reviews — A combination of studies on a specific topic

Level 2 — Evidence syntheses — Critically appraised papers that inform the reader about the strength of the evidence

Level 3 — Article synopses — Critical appraisal and evaluation of a single research study

Level 4 — Randomised controlled trials

Level 5 — Cohort studies — Observational studies of groups but these cannot determine if an intervention is effective

Level 6 — Case studies and reports

Level 7 (least reliable evidence) — Opinions, editorials and anecdotes

Figure 7.1 *The hierarchy of evidence.*

ACTIVITY 7.4

Select a journal that you have read to keep up to date or used to gain information for an assignment. Check the list of contents to see if you can find research reports and other types of articles that mirror some of the levels of evidence in the hierarchy for EBP shown in *Fig. 7.1*. Consider how published articles can help inform practice but be critical in your reading and thinking; an 'Editorial' may be expert opinion but can also be a contemporary version of 'Sister says'.

FURTHER READING

Critical appraisal checklists. Available at: https://casp-uk.net/casp-tools-checklists (accessed 2 December 2022).

Evidence-based nursing resources. Available at: https://s4be.cochrane.org/blog/2017/03/09/library-evidence-based-nursing-resources or bit.ly/3kBf4HW (accessed 2 December 2022).

Heaslip, V. and Lindsay, B. (2019) *Research and Evidence-based Practice: for nursing, health and social care students.* Lantern Publishing.

References

Grove, S.K., Gray, J.R. and Burns, N. (2015) *Understanding Nursing Research: building an evidence-based practice*, 6th edition. Saunders.

Guest, J.F., Singh, H., Rana, K. and Vowden, P. (2018) Cost-effectiveness of an electroceutical device in treating non-healing venous leg ulcers: results of an RCT. *Journal of Wound Care*, **27**(4): 230–243.

Hopkins, A. (2004) Disrupted lives: investigating coping strategies for non-healing leg ulcers. *British Journal of Nursing*, **13**(9): 556–563.

Lagerin, A., Hylander, I. and Törnkvist, L. (2017) District nurses' experiences of caring for leg ulcers in accordance with clinical guidelines: a grounded theory study. *International Journal of Qualitative Studies on Health and Wellbeing*, **12**(1): 1355213.

Lauzon Clabo, L.M. (2007) An ethnography of pain assessment and the role of social context on two postoperative units. *Journal of Advanced Nursing*, **61**(5): 531–539.

Leren, L., Johansen, E.A., Eide, H., Sørum Falk, R. and Ljoså, T.M. (2021) Prevalence and factors associated with ulcer-related pain in persons with chronic leg ulcers – an explorative study. *Journal of Clinical Nursing*, **30**(3): 2732–2741.

Lindsay, E. (2018) Monitoring service quality: Lindsay Leg Club member satisfaction survey. *British Journal of Community Nursing Supplement*, **23**(Sup12): S24–S28.

Jolley, J. (2020) *Introducing Research and Evidence-Based Practice for Nursing and Healthcare Professionals*, 3rd edition. Routledge.

Lernevall, L., Fogh, K., Nielsen, C., Dam, W. and Dreyer, P. (2017) Lived experiences of life with a leg ulcer – a life in hell. *European Wound Management Association Journal*, **17**(1): 15–21.

Minyan Zhao, B.S., Dongting Zhang, B.S., Liping Tan, M.D. and Hui Huang, M.D. (2020) Silver dressings for the healing of venous leg ulcer: a meta-analysis and systematic review. *Medicine*, 99(37): 1–9.

NMC (2018) *Standards of Proficiency for Nursing Associates*. Nursing and Midwifery Council.

Porter-O'Grady, T. (2006) 'A new age for practice: creating the framework for evidence'. In Malloch, K. and Porter-O'Grady, T. (eds) *Introduction to Evidence-based Practice in Nursing and Health Care* (pp. 1–29). Jones and Bartlett.

Probst, S., Bobbink, P., Séchaud, L. and Buehrer Skinner, M. (2021) Venous leg ulcer recurrences – the relationship to self-efficacy, social support and quality of life – a mixed method study. *Journal of Advanced Nursing*, 77(1): 367–375.

Rees, A., Beecroft, C. and Booth, A. (2015) 'Critical appraisal of the evidence'. In Gerrish, K. and Lathlean, J. (eds) *The Research Process in Nursing*, 7th edition. Wiley-Blackwell.

Schmidt, N.A. and Brown, J.M. (2019) *Evidence-based Practice for Nurses: appraisal and application of research*. Jones & Bartlett.

Wong, M.M-K., Chong, H.-M., Chun, N. and Yap, J.C.-M. (2020) Transcutaneous electrical nerve stimulation to treat pain in patients with venous leg ulceration. *Wounds International*, **11**(3): 30–33.

Ylonen, M., Viljamaa, J., Isoaho, H. *et al.* (2017) Internet-based learning programme to increase nurses' knowledge level about venous leg ulcer care in home health care. *Journal of Clinical Nursing*, **26**(21–22): 3646–3657.

MENTAL HEALTH

David Matthews

This chapter relates to outcomes 2.2, 2.3, 2.5, 2.6, 3.1, 3.2, 3.3 and 3.19 within the *Standards of Proficiency for Nursing Associates* (NMC, 2018).

LEARNING OUTCOMES

When you have completed this chapter you should be able to:
- Define mental health and mental illness.
- Outline the concept of mental health.
- Appreciate different disciplinary understandings of mental health.
- Appreciate the broad understandings of mental health conditions.
- Develop awareness of an evidence-based approach to the treatment of mental health problems.
- Increase your knowledge of service delivery linked to NICE guidance.

8.1 Introduction

The purpose of this chapter is to explore the concept of mental health. An attempt will be made to define what is meant by mental health and similar concepts, as various terms are used by health professionals when discussing mental health. Additionally possible causes of mental health problems will be discussed by exploring various theoretical understandings, with a brief overview of biological, psychological and sociological factors. Moreover, some of the most common mental health diagnoses will be investigated, and an overview of the services and provision available will be provided.

8.2 What do we mean by 'mental health'?

Mental illness, as a concept, has been in existence since antiquity. Throughout history, including up to many of our lifetimes, varying derogatory terms have been used to describe mental illness and those living with poor mental health, such as 'lunacy', 'insanity', 'crazy', 'psycho', 'nutter', 'insane' and many more. In the seventeenth and eighteenth centuries experts in the mental health field were known as 'alienists' due to the sense that they were managing other-worldly behaviours and presentations. Consequently, the madhouses of this era often used experimental methods without the ethical approval required in today's modern healthcare services. So, it seems that since ancient times those who have presented with behaviours and beliefs which sit outside of social norms and expectations have been viewed as different and in some cases considered 'insane' or mentally ill. Recent decades, however, have arguably witnessed an increasing change in attitude.

Since 1992, 10 October has been World Mental Health Day, being an effort to raise awareness of mental health globally. Combined with a growing number of health promotion campaigns in many countries, including the UK, focusing on promoting good mental health, it is clear that the last few decades have witnessed an increasing focus upon, and acceptance of the importance of, positive mental health for individuals. However, despite this, mental health remains an elusive concept to define. Since the early 2000s, the World Health Organization (WHO, 2004, p. 12) has defined mental health as "a state of wellbeing in which the individual realizes his or her own abilities, can cope with the normal stresses of life, can work productively and fruitfully, and is able to make a contribution to his or her community".

ACTIVITY 8.1

Think about the definition of mental health produced by the WHO. Based on this, what do you think an individual needs to achieve good mental health?

Despite the popularity of the WHO's definition, there is no agreed-upon understanding of mental health. This lack of consensus is illustrated in popular culture; for example, the novel and film *One Flew Over the Cuckoo's Nest*, and films such as *A Beautiful Mind* starring Russell Crowe, *Black Swan* starring Natalie Portman and *Split* starring James McAvoy, have all tried to portray the experiences of someone with mental health problems. While these may be useful resources to help us gain some insights and understanding, mental health has been portrayed in varying ways.

ACTIVITY 8.2

In what ways is mental health portrayed in the media and popular culture?

8.2.1 Mental wellbeing

For Dave, Jenkins and Dogra (2016) the term 'mental health' is best understood as referring to a spectrum of experiences, ranging from positive to negative. Mental health, they argue, is a status referring to an individual's mental wellbeing at any point in time in their lives, with it being the case that we may experience good or poor mental health and wellbeing at any time. A mental health status is something that we all have at all times, as mental health is something which everyone has. Positive mental wellbeing is a sense of equilibrium. This means a sense of balance in life and calm state of mind which allows a person to be able to achieve activities of daily living effectively. This usually involves having some sense of achievement and effective outcome to the day.

8.2.2 Mental health problems

The experience of poor mental health gives rise to the concept of 'mental health problems'. This can often refer to problems which are mild but which nevertheless impact upon an individual's daily functioning (Dave, Jenkins and Dogra, 2016). The breakdown of a relationship, a bereavement, moving to a new area where you do not know anyone, a change of job, or increased responsibilities at work, can all potentially have a negative impact on our mental health, resulting in us experiencing feelings of loneliness, anxiety, isolation and depression.

Mental health problems can arise in response to certain triggers and our own interpretations of surrounding environments and situations. If a person is feeling mentally well, they tend to cope more effectively with life stressors and have an ability to problem-solve more effectively. Achieving and maintaining wellbeing involves remaining physically active, socialising with others, learning new skills such as cooking a new recipe or starting a new hobby, giving to others as this creates a sense of purpose and self-worth, and being able to focus in the present moment. It is ultimately all about creating the balance between the pressures and more mundane aspects of life and the more rewarding pleasurable aspects of life.

When a person becomes mentally unwell, they have generally lost balance, and this can be caused by a variety of reasons that will be discussed later in the chapter. The person who is not feeling as well tends to struggle with problem-solving or makes rash decisions which can be counterproductive and create more stressors. For example, drinking more alcohol can relax some people but in other cases, drinking excessively can lead to drunken arguments or severe hangovers which then add to the cycle of low mood and self-critical thoughts.

While mental health problems are troublesome for us at the time, such experiences do not necessarily mean that we have a mental illness. It is quite possible to have poor mental health but not have a mental illness.

8.2.3 Mental illness

According to the American Psychiatric Association (2022), "Mental illnesses are health conditions involving changes in emotion, thinking or behaviour (or a combination of these). Mental illnesses are associated with distress and/or problems functioning in social, work or family activities". Strongly associated with the term 'mental illness', and often used interchangeably, is that of 'mental disorder'. Mental illnesses and mental disorders are, Dave, Jenkins and Dogra (2016) assert, disturbances of thinking, perception and behaviours which cannot be considered developmentally appropriate, and potentially interfere with an individual's ability to engage with everyday expectations. The terms mental illness and mental disorder are commonly mental health problems that fit diagnostic criteria, and thus an individual can be said to have a mental illness or mental disturbance if they have been exposed to the diagnostic process and come into contact with mental health professionals.

8.3 Stigma

The actual rate of mental illness, and more broadly mental health problems, is difficult to identify, in the UK as in many other countries. In part, this is as a consequence of under-reporting. Moreover, unlike physical health issues, which physically manifest themselves, mental health issues cannot be easily identified. Their diagnosis often relies upon mental health professionals interpreting the actions and emotional conditions of individuals based upon a set of criteria which are understood as indicating the existence of a mental illness. However, that said, efforts to measure the predominance of mental health issues have revealed they are prevalent within the population. In 2021 in England an estimated 1 in 6 adults experienced, in any week, a common mental health disorder such as depression, anxiety, panic disorders and obsessive–compulsive disorder (Baker, 2021). Moreover, globally, the WHO (2022) asserts that depression is one of the main causes of disability. Furthermore, they also report that suicide is the fourth leading cause of death among those aged 15–29 years, with 700,000 people of all ages dying every year due to suicide, with many of these having never had any contact with mental health services (WHO, 2022).

Despite its prevalence, mental illness remains stigmatised. For the sociologist Goffman (1990[1963]), stigma referred to an attribute held by an individual which was socially discredited, with individuals thus stigmatised failing to gain social acceptance. A historian of mental illness, Porter (2013), argues that stigmatisation involves identifying understood differences of the stigmatised group, invoking society's fear of them, and making explicit a perception of their inferiority justifying discriminatory treatment. Those with mental health issues have for centuries been stigmatised. As a result of fear and prejudice, strict confinement and regulation characterised their historic treatment, in an effort to separate the 'normal' from the 'mad' (Porter, 2013). While undoubtedly attitudes have become more accepting and favourable to individuals with mental health issues, mental illness remains stigmatised in British society.

ACTIVITY 8.3

Think of examples of how individuals with mental health problems are stigmatised in society.

Individuals with mental illness continue to experience stigma and discrimination in all aspects of their lives. In some cases, individuals will not seek help when they are struggling with mental health problems as it is not recognised as an issue within their culture, as can sometimes be the case among some cultural groups in the UK, or frowned upon and seen as a sign of weakness, as has commonly been argued to be the case among men. There can also be stereotypical views of mental illness, such as believing people with mental health issues are dangerous and a risk to others, which has created a sense of fear amongst the public. This is fuelled by media coverage of incidents which have involved murder or criminal activity. If an individual had a physical concern such as diabetes or heart disease, they would seek medical attention and appropriate treatment, but this is often not the case when a person is struggling with mental health problems. In many cases leaning on self-medication such as alcohol, street drugs or analgesic medications is preferred and seen as less stigmatising.

Social media can have a positive and negative impact on mental health. There have been some useful campaigns to help raise awareness; examples include:

- Heads Together: a mental health initiative led by the Royal Foundation of the Prince and Princess of Wales, the aim being to tackle stigma and change society's views on mental health with fundraising and other training (www.headstogether.org.uk).
- #Hereforyou: an Instagram-based campaign aimed at encouraging people to share their stories and support each other (www.instagram.com/explore/tags/hereforyou).
- UOKM8?: an initiative launched by the LADbible group which aims to reach out to men (www.ladbible.com/uokm8). This was inspired by data suggesting the highest killer in men under 45 is suicide.
- Time to Change: a campaign led by the charities Mind and Rethink Mental Illness that ran from 2007 to 2021 (www.time-to-change.org.uk). Positive

outcomes were reported following the campaign, with 1.2 million people changing attitudes to mental health since 2016 and discrimination in employment and on a societal level falling, according to the campaign's 2016–2021 impact report.

8.4 Labelling

As a consequence of the stigma associated with mental health issues, a diagnosis of a mental illness can lead to an individual being labelled as having a mental illness. This can have negative consequences for the individual in question, especially if it becomes publicly known that the person has been diagnosed.

The stigmatisation of mental illness is a reflection of the continuing broad belief in society that mental illness is a form of deviancy, in that the behaviours and emotional condition of those with a mental illness are opposed to what is considered accepted behaviour and emotions. As sociologist Becker (2018[1963]) argued in his classic study, there are certain behaviours, actions and feelings which society labels as deviant, including criminality, some physical conditions and mental illness. For many exponents of labelling theory, there is nothing inherent in many of the actions and feelings which make them deviant. Rather, society has chosen to identify them as deviant, as they are in opposition to what society has decided as acceptable actions and feelings (Morrall, 2009). With regard to mental illness, while not disputing the existence of mental health problems generally, there has been a history of social scientists and critical/radical psychiatrists who have argued that a considerable amount of the behaviour, actions, thoughts and feelings identified as mental illness is in fact not an example of existing mental health issues, but instead society arguing that these forms of behaviours and thoughts are 'abnormal'.

» **There is a risk that the label of mental illness overrides all other aspects of an individual's identity and becomes the primary label that defines them.**

Being labelled as having a mental illness is a powerful social label, but its influence can only materialise if the label is imposed by someone who has the professional and social status to do so. An individual being called mentally ill in a pub after a heated exchange or argument is unlikely to experience the consequences of the label. However, that same individual accessing mental health services and being exposed to the interventions of mental health professionals and subject to diagnosis, resulting in being labelled as having a mental illness, is more likely to experience negative consequences of this label. Being thrust upon them by mental health professionals who are accepted by society as having the authority to intervene in the lives of individuals, the label is likely to be accepted by the wider public and society.

ACTIVITY 8.4

Why do mental health professionals have the ability and authority to label someone as having a mental health problem?

When a label as dominant as mental illness is given to someone by those who have the authority to do so, it often becomes a lens through which others view that individual. Their behaviour, thoughts and feelings can be interpreted, by both health professionals and members of the public, as reflecting and confirming the label of mental illness. There exists the danger that the label of mental illness becomes an individual's master status, with this label overriding all other aspects of an individual's identity and becoming the primary label that defines them. Moreover, the individual who is labelled as being mentally ill may internalise that label, and all that is associated with it, and subsequently come to understand themselves through the lens of that label. Individuals may begin to act in accordance with the expectations of the label and society's expectations of someone who has that label. The result is a self-fulfilling prophecy (Goodman, 2015).

8.5 Mental health problems: biological, psychological and sociological causes

The causes of mental health issues are varied. As professionals from different backgrounds compete with each other to have their understandings of the causes accepted, there is no agreed definitive understanding. Overall, however, the majority of explanations can be roughly divided into the areas of biological, psychological and sociological causes.

8.5.1 Biological

Reflecting the dominance of the biomedical model within healthcare generally, biological explanations for mental health issues are arguably some of the most influential. The biological view is based on the premise that a physical cause can be found to explain the symptoms presented. Psychiatry encapsulates this approach to mental health in accepting a medical understanding, engaging in the diagnosis of poor mental health, and attempting to identify the cause of mental illness and sufficient medical interventions as treatment. Medicines and drugs are seized upon as being largely the preferred method of treatment.

The popularity and subsequent dominance of this biological model of mental illness can be illustrated with reference to the dopamine hypothesis, also known as the 'chemical imbalance' theory, which suggests that schizophrenia is caused by an overactivity of dopamine systems. Likewise, it is suggested that depleted neurotransmitter levels or a reduction in the number of serotonin receptors can lead to depression. However, Cromby *et al.* (2013) suggest that it is difficult to find reliable research supporting these theories and inconsistencies are found; for example, not all individuals with schizophrenia have an excess of dopamine.

Over recent decades there have been advances in genetics and neuroscience which have helped to increase understanding of the biological nature of mental health problems. Also, newer psychotropic medications have become available with fewer side-effects, which have seemingly been beneficial in the management of some mental health disorders (Angermeyer *et al.*, 2018). There has also been extensive research into genetic causes for mental health problems, but again this is not conclusive as there are various complexities and variables in the research outcomes. As a result, mental health assessments are generally based on interviews and observations which include self-reports of a person's experiences and symptoms. Currently, there are no specific blood tests or scans which can confirm specific mental health diagnoses. Even in cases of dementia, brain scans do not always show brain abnormalities but can be useful in determining other causes or types of dementia. Research has been conducted into links between mental health problems and autoimmune disorders, as discussed by Mehta (2020); it is suggested there is an overlap in symptoms, and one may lead to another. Using a more transdiagnostic approach in this area may be more beneficial to patients, as antidepressants have been reported to have some anti-inflammatory benefits and anti-inflammatory medications seem to have some antidepressant effect.

A fundamental criticism of the psychiatric understanding of mental illness is that, in the main, it deals with symptoms and their treatment, rather than causes. While arguing that biology plays a significant role, psychiatry largely concedes that mental illness is frequently not visible, only its impact upon individuals in the form of symptoms. Therefore, we can conclude that while biological factors should not be ruled out as influencing the development of mental health issues, there may not always be enough evidence to say this is a primary cause in all cases (Davies, 2013; Harrington, 2019). Biological factors need to be considered alongside psychological social factors to ensure a more rounded holistic approach.

8.5.2 Psychological

The psychological approach suggests that the cause of mental health problems is a consequence of the individuals' reactions to life stressors and experiences. This perspective suggests that problems often develop due to a person's beliefs about a situation, focusing on cycles and patterns of thoughts, feelings and behaviours. In particular, psychological approaches emphasise issues of normality and abnormality.

Psychology's attempts to adopt the methods and practices of the natural sciences, engaging in research and experiments and accepting the use of quantitative data, as Rogers and Pilgrim (2021) argue, have resulted in psychology trying to ascertain the normality or abnormality of behaviours by determining their frequency in the population. As professionals, psychologists attempt to identify the extent to which characteristics are commonplace or not within a population, attempting to determine the statistical prevalence of mental health issues and the chances of individuals acquiring them. Such an approach is common within abnormal psychology and clinical psychology.

In its pursuit of exemplifying the normal and abnormal, psychology attempts to identify developmental norms, with such approaches as cognitive psychology constructing and offering a framework against which to measure developmental expectations. Moreover, psychological perspectives, such as humanistic psychology, measure mental health against an ideal notion of what human development should be, and be characterised by. Optimal mental health is identified if an individual is able to achieve personal fulfilment. Poor mental health, it is argued, may arise from experiencing any impediment in an individual's psychological development.

8.5.3 Sociological

A sociological understanding of mental health problems has been considered since the early nineteenth century. Dominant within this approach has been a social causation perspective. Mental health issues, while being considered a real biological issue which impacts upon the body, are largely deemed to have their origins not in the physical and biological nature of the individual, but rather in the wider social context and society within which the individual lives and works. A social cause is identified, with issues such as poverty, crime, unemployment, housing conditions, racism and discrimination, sexism and employment conditions, identified as having the potential to impact negatively upon an individual's mental wellbeing (Rogers and Pilgrim, 2021). Within a sociological approach, as Rogers and Pilgrim (2021) assert, there is often an attempt to identify the relationship between social disadvantage and mental illness.

Economic circumstances

While anyone, regardless of their background, has a chance of developing poor mental health, sociological studies have illustrated that not everyone has the same chance, with some individuals more likely than others. As with physical health more generally, sociological investigations have identified the extent to which poverty and low income determine someone's chances of developing a mental illness, with evidence indicating that the poorer an individual is, the more likely they are to experience negative mental wellbeing (Matthews, 2019). Low income and its consequences, such as financial insecurity, inability to afford necessities and poor housing, can have serious consequences, encouraging anxiety and depression, as well as substance abuse. In a similar vein, Warner (2004) identified the relationship between poorer economic circumstances and the development of schizophrenia. That there is a strong relationship between an individual's economic circumstances and mental health can be illustrated by the fact that in England the most recent evidence reported in 2021 identified that 33% of economically inactive people – individuals who are either unemployed or not looking for work – reported having mental health issues such as anxiety and depression, compared to 14% who were in full-time employment (Baker, 2021).

Gender

Gender is also considered as an important factor under the sociological perspective. Pilgrim and McKeown (2018) state that there is a higher level of diagnosis of depression in women in the primary care setting. This could be explained by more females presenting for appointments in primary care as opposed to males or, Pilgrim and McKeown (2018) suggest, that women could be more oppressed than males. Consequently, there exists some controversy regarding these debates, but data does suggest the gender differences and link to mental health problems require some acknowledgement. The expectations of gender roles in society may also contribute to this discussion, and the creation of stereotype behaviours can lead to a pressure to behave or perform in certain ways.

Ethnicity

In terms of ethnicity, again social patterns emerge. Overall, individuals from ethnic minority backgrounds have a greater chance of experiencing poorer mental health compared to those from the white ethnic majority population in the UK. Reasons for this are complex and varied, but include experiencing prejudicial attitudes by service providers, by health and social care organisations and by the state more generally, greater chance of being exposed to social causes of mental illness such as poverty and unemployment, the stress of adjusting to a new life and culture if recently having migrated to the UK, and being victims of more general racism and discrimination in society (Barry and Yuill, 2016). That ethnic groups have varying chances of experiencing poor mental health can again be illustrated statistically with evidence published in 2021, for England, indicating that 23% of Black British individuals were likely to report experiencing anxiety and depression compared to 17% of White British (Baker, 2021).

ACTIVITY 8.5

Think about someone who works in a low paid job which is insecure. How might that impact upon their mental health?

The sociological perspective emphasises the importance of allowing service users to have power and control over their own care, ensuring the best decisions are made for them by them. Awareness of stigmatisation and discrimination is an important aspect of this approach to care. This can conflict in view with the medical model which is more focused on the traditional doctor–patient relationship based on the understanding that the doctor has the expertise and is seen as holding a powerful position, in contrast to the patient who is more passive and has little choice (Golightley and Goemans, 2017).

Although there remains great debate as to the causes of mental illness, especially with regard to biological arguments, a position which is increasingly becoming accepted is to acknowledge the relationship between society and biology. The individual is a biological entity, but one positioned within a social context, with it being difficult to separate the two. Social experiences have direct consequences for our physiology, including that related to our mental wellbeing, and biological change can contribute to poor mental wellbeing as a consequence of being influenced by social determinants and experiences.

RECAP

- Mental health may be best understood as a spectrum of experiences, ranging from positive to negative.
- Mental illness and mental disorder are commonly understood as mental health problems that fit certain diagnostic criteria.
- Despite the prevalence of mental illness, individuals with mental illness experience stigma and discrimination.
- The causes of mental health issues are varied, but the majority of explanations can be roughly divided into the areas of biological, psychological and sociological causes.

8.6 Mental health across the life course

It has been illustrated that poor mental health is not evenly distributed within the population, with different social groups at greater risk of experiencing it than others. Gender, ethnicity and low economic status are significant determinants. In addition to these variables, age plays an influential role, with the chances of experiencing poor mental health varying across the life course

>> **An individual's chances of experiencing poor mental wellbeing will differ at varying points in their life depending upon their circumstances and experiences at the time.**

(Larkin, 2013). Although attempts to ascertain the rate of mental illness can be challenging, there exists a broad understanding that rates are greatest among younger age groups and the oldest with, Larkin (2013) argues, a broad U-shape pattern characterising the distribution of mental illness across the life course.

8.6.1 Children and young people

Research in 2020 by Unicef clearly stated that relative to many other countries the mental wellbeing of British children was poor, with the UK ranked 29 out of 38 countries when the life satisfaction of 15-year-olds was taken into account as well as suicide rates among those aged 15–19 years (Unicef, 2020). Furthermore, evidence for England in 2021 indicated that mental health disorders were common among 17.4% of all those aged 6–16 years, compared to 11.6% in 2017. Very similar figures applied to those aged 17–19 years. Among children aged 6–10 years, boys were far more likely to experience mental health problems, whereas between 11 and 16 years old the trend was for girls to experience a greater prevalence (Baker, 2021).

Of significant consequence for a child's mental health are what are referred to as Adverse Childhood Experiences (ACEs), which are identified as highly stressful and traumatic experiences which happen during childhood. According to Petruccelli, Davis and Berman (2019), they have been found to have a significant impact on an individual's development and future physical and mental health, impacting upon them not just in childhood, but later in life as well.

> **ACTIVITY 8.6**
>
> What do you think constitutes an adverse childhood experience which would impact upon a child's mental health?

While recognising that poor mental wellbeing is an experience that many children and young people suffer, it is arguably the case that a significant proportion of mental health problems among this age group are not recognised. As a consequence, young children in particular are subsequently at greater risk later in life of experiencing further mental health issues (Larkin, 2013). Commonly, if undiagnosed in childhood, mental health issues are likely to manifest and become most visible during adolescence and early adulthood, with three-quarters of all mental illnesses having begun by the mid-20s. Typical mental health disorders during this period in the life course include obsessive–compulsive disorder and eating disorders.

ACTIVITY 8.7

What risk factors exist during adolescence which increase the possible onset of mental health issues at this point in an individual's life?

8.6.2 People in midlife

Advancing towards and entering midlife, the risk of developing mental health issues subsides, yet risks remain. Relationships play a significant role in influencing the development of poor mental wellbeing during this period. Midlife is a period where there is an increased risk of long-term relationships breaking down. Individuals who are single are less likely to report feeling happy, with those being married experiencing greater levels of satisfaction and being at less risk of depression. The experience of divorce in this period of an individual's life exposes them to increased risk of stress, depression, anxiety and substance abuse. Moreover, as relationships break down new ones are often created. The process of marrying again, becoming a step-parent, and children from different relationships coming together as one new family, can be both challenging and stressful.

8.6.3 Older people

In old age, again an individual's circumstances specific to this period within their life course can have detrimental consequences for their mental health. Becoming widowed characterises the lives of many in old age, a potential consequence of which can be the experience of significant grief and a sense of isolation and loneliness. Increased alcohol consumption has been identified as a possible mechanism for coping with losing a spouse, and depression can be another consequence. However, as Larkin (2013) argues, while women are more likely to be widowed because they tend to live longer than men, women on the whole cope better with this loss than men, as they are more likely to have a wider social network than men.

A further significant challenge to mental wellbeing in old age is that of continuing caring responsibilities. For women in particular, caring for another individual is something that characterises the lives of many during varying periods across their life course, from children in their younger years, to elderly parents during middle age, and then caring for a partner in old age. Whether a man or a woman, however, being a carer in old age can be detrimental to mental health. Caring for an elderly partner may require a level of care which is intensive, given the potential needs and conditions an elderly partner may have, such as dementia.

Moreover, an elderly carer has a higher chance of also experiencing health issues themselves, with the need to cope with this and at the same time support an elderly partner being potentially very challenging for them. Additionally, in this period in an individual's life, it is not just elderly partners that older individuals may find themselves supporting. With childcare costs absorbing a large proportion of parents' monthly income, and the almost universal expectation that women will enter the labour force, many grandparents have taken on the responsibility for the care of grandchildren. Such support has been identified as contributing to increasing poor mental wellbeing among older individuals, exacerbating feelings of stress (Lee and Jang, 2019).

Recognition of how mental wellbeing may vary across the life course is to accept that an individual's chances of experiencing poor mental wellbeing will differ at varying points in their life depending upon their circumstances and experiences at the time. Age must be accepted as a determinant of mental wellbeing, but it does not operate independently of those factors which we have already discussed. The chances of an individual experiencing mental health issues at various periods throughout their life course are dependent on the interaction between sociological, psychological and biological factors at particular points throughout the life course.

8.7 Mental health conditions

As a nursing associate you are likely to come into contact with individuals of varying states of mental wellbeing and who display a variety of mental health issues. Although it is not possible to provide an exhaustive list, the purpose here is to present a brief introduction and overview of some of the more common mental health disorders you are likely to be presented with. As already indicated above, evidence from 2021 for England indicated that one in six adults above the age of sixteen reported experiencing a mental health issue in any given week.

8.7.1 Generalised anxiety disorder (GAD)

Evidence for England suggests that GAD is the most commonly experienced mental health issue (Baker, 2021). Symptoms primarily include excessive anxiety and worrying about different activities and events, occurring more days than not for at least six months. The person may find this difficult to control. Other symptoms can include feeling restless, irritable or fatigued, muscle tension, sleeping difficulty and difficulty concentrating. The individual usually experiences a significant amount of distress and impairment in many areas of functioning because of these symptoms.

>> **GAD is the most-experienced mental health disorder in England.**

8.7.2 Depression

Depression is a common and well-known mental health condition, being the second most widely reported mental health issue in 2021 in England (Baker, 2021). It is generally recognised by reports or observations of low mood and feelings of sadness, emptiness and hopelessness. The individual with depression can experience tearfulness and notice a reduction in enjoyment or pleasure in daily activities. A person can experience weight loss or gain due to reduction or increase in appetite. Sleep disturbance is also a common symptom leading to feelings of tiredness. In some cases, this can lead to a sense of being slowed down which may be observable to others.

Depression is usually accompanied by negative thinking and self-critical thoughts including a sense of guilt and shame, alongside an inability to concentrate or make decisions. In some severe cases thoughts of suicide can be evident. As with all mental health conditions individual presentations are on a continuum from mild to severe, and patients should be assessed and treatment planned accordingly.

8.7.3 Obsessive–compulsive disorder

Obsessive–compulsive disorder (OCD) is characterised by the presence of either obsessions or compulsions. An obsession is an unwelcome thought or image which is unwanted and causes distress. The individual will make attempts to suppress or ignore the obsessions, but this is largely unsuccessful. Compulsions are repetitive behaviours or mental acts such as hand washing, counting or praying with the subconscious aim of relieving anxiety and uncomfortable feelings.

Obsessions and compulsions are time-consuming and can take more than one hour per day, causing significant impact on the person's daily functioning. An important note to make is that many people talk about having OCD, but this may not meet the

>> OCD can have significant consequences for the functioning of an individual on an everyday basis.

full diagnostic criteria if it does not cause a significant impact on their daily functioning. It has in fact become a popular trend to say "my OCD". We all have certain ritualistic behaviours which we follow. This is normal human behaviour and some of it is repetitive in nature and keeps us functioning well, such as a routine of washing and dressing. However, those who meet the diagnostic criteria for OCD tend to have an inflated sense of responsibility linked to the safety of others and a tendency to overestimate the threat in certain situations, which leads to an increase in the intensity of rituals and checking behaviours.

8.7.4 Phobia

A phobia is recognised as a specific fear or anxiety about a situation or specific object. This might include things like spiders, lifts, clowns, dogs, mice and seeing blood. The diagnostic criteria emphasise that these objects or situations always provoke intense fear and anxiety. The person usually actively avoids the phobic situation or will endure it with intense fear. This fear is persistent and avoided where possible and to meet the diagnostic criteria it needs to be present for longer than six months.

8.7.5 Panic disorder

The main symptoms of panic disorder are unexpected panic attacks which can occur abruptly, creating an intense fear and discomfort which can peak very quickly.

Panic disorder symptoms can include the following:
- Palpitations
- Trembling and shaking
- Sweating and hot flushes or chills and shivering
- A dry mouth, shortness of breath or choking sensation
- Nausea, dizziness and feeling faint
- Numbness, pins and needles or a tingling sensation
- Chest pain
- A churning stomach
- Feeling detached from yourself, losing control or 'going crazy'.

The person experiencing panic attacks also has a persistent worry about future panic attacks and has usually developed some behaviours to avoid having panic attacks such as using the stairs rather than going in a lift, if using a lift would induce a panic attack.

8.8 Intervention and support

Reflecting the complexity of debates as to what causes poor mental health, there exist varying methods of support and interventions. When considering treatment options for individuals presenting with mental health problems, it is important that an evidence-based practice approach is used. The National Institute for Health and Care Excellence (NICE) provides a variety of guidance documents that are appropriate to the delivery of treatments for mental health conditions (see *Table 8.1*). The guidance recommends that a stepped care model is followed in terms of finding the most appropriate service for an individual presenting with potential mental health problems. This ranges from someone going to see their GP with mild low mood/anxiety to someone who presents with psychotic-type symptoms and is assessed by a crisis team.

As highlighted previously, the approach to mental health care has changed dramatically over the years, moving from institutionalised care to a focus on community-based care and a preventative approach. The introduction of more effective mental health specific medications from the 1950s onwards, such as the expansion of antidepressants reflecting the dominance of the medical model, and then a move to more psychological interventions such as cognitive behavioural therapy (CBT) in the last fifteen years, has transformed the way care is delivered. This approach has allowed for a broader reach of service provision. According to the National Collaborating Centre for Mental Health (2021) over 1.15 million people gained access to services in 2019/20. Some of the interventions available are delivered quickly and in a short time frame but have effective outcomes on patient wellbeing and recovery rates. The NHS Long Term Plan (NHS England, 2019) emphasised the expansion of primary care improving access to psychological therapies to ensure 1.9 million people per year can access services by 2023/24.

Mental health services are also developing a more trauma-informed approach to mental health care which involves recognising that a high proportion of individuals accessing mental health services at any level have experienced some level of trauma in their lives that has not been acknowledged before. This means that care delivery has previously been focused on the reduction of symptoms but not on the reason for the problem. Dawson *et al.* (2021) have commenced a review of studies related to trauma-informed care approaches in community and primary care services, and this has been identified in the NHS Long Term Plan (2019). The aim of this review is to work towards a model of service delivery incorporating the trauma-informed angle.

Table 8.1 *NICE-recommended psychological interventions (adapted from National Collaborating Centre for Mental Health, 2021)*

	Condition	Psychological therapy option	Source
Step 1 treatment	Minimum symptoms of anxiety or low mood	Watchful waiting under GP care Recognising problem area	
Step 2 treatment: low intensity interventions	Depression	Individual guided self-help based on CBT, computerised CBT, behavioural activation, structured group physical activity programme	NICE guidelines: CG90, CG91, CG123
	Generalised anxiety disorder	Self-help, or guided self-help, based on CBT, psycho-educational groups, computerised CBT	NICE guidelines: CG113, CG123
	Panic disorder	Self-help, or guided self-help, based on CBT, psycho-educational groups, computerised CBT	NICE guidelines: CG113, CG123
	Obsessive–compulsive disorder	Guided self-help based on CBT	NICE guidelines: CG31, CG123

Table 8.1 (continued)

	Condition	Psychological therapy option	Source
Step 3: high intensity interventions	Depression For individuals with mild–moderate severity who have not responded to initial low intensity interventions	CBT (individual or group) or IPT Behavioural activation Couples therapy Counselling for depression Brief psychodynamic therapy **Note:** psychological interventions can be provided in combination with anti-depressant medication	NICE guidelines: CG90, CG91, CG123
	Depression Moderate–severe	CBT (individual) or IPT, each with medication CBT or mindfulness-based cognitive therapy	NICE guidelines: CG113, CG123
	Generalised anxiety disorder	CBT, applied relaxation	NICE guidelines: CG113, CG123
	Panic disorder	CBT	NICE guidelines: CG113, CG123
	PTSD	Trauma-focused CBT, eye movement desensitisation and reprocessing	NICE guidelines: NG116
	Social anxiety disorder	CBT specific for social anxiety disorder	NICE guideline: CG159
	OCD	CBT (including exposure and response prevention)	NICE guidelines: CG31, CG123

CHAPTER SUMMARY

- Positive mental wellbeing equates to a balance in life, providing a sense of achievement for the individual and self-worth.
- Mental health problems can be triggered by life events and a change in our circumstances and/or our interpretation of these.
- Although more widely discussed, mental illness still carries a stigma which can make sufferers reluctant to seek help.

- Poor mental health is not evenly spread across the population. Gender, ethnicity and low economic status all influence the distribution. Rates are higher in younger and older members of society.
- Biological, psychological and sociological factors are offered as causative factors for mental illness, but there is no agreed definitive understanding.

FURTHER READING

Chadwick, A. and Murphy, N. (2021) *Mental Health: a non-specialist introduction for nursing and health care.* Lantern Publishing.

Cromby, J., Harper, D. and Reavey. P. (2013) *Psychology, Mental Health and Distress.* Palgrave Macmillan.

Golightley, M. and Goemans, R. (2017) *Social Work and Mental Health*, 6th edition. Sage.

Rogers, A. and Pilgrim, D. (2021) *A Sociology of Mental Health and Illness*, 6th edition. Open University Press.

References

American Psychiatric Association (2022) *What is Mental Illness?* Available at: www.psychiatry.org/patients-families/what-is-mental-illness or bit.ly/3SIdRLq (accessed 5 December 2022).

Angermeyer, M., Matschinge, H. and Schomerus, G. (2018) Attitudes towards psychiatric treatment and people with mental illness: changes over two decades. *The British Journal of Psychiatry*, **203**(2): 146–151.

Baker, C. (2021) *Mental Health Statistics England.* Available at: https://commonslibrary.parliament.uk/research-briefings/sn06988/#:~:text=A%202021%20survey%20of%20children,similar%20between%202020%20and%202021 or bit.ly/3KU4Yg2 (accessed 5 December 2022).

Barry, A. and Yuill, C. (2016) *Understanding the Sociology of Health*, 4th edition. Sage.

Becker, H. (2018[1963]) *Outsiders: Studies in the sociology of deviance.* Free Press.

Cromby, J., Harper, D. and Reavey. P. (2013) *Psychology, Mental Health and Distress.* Palgrave Macmillan.

Dave, S., Jenkins, R. and Dogra, N. (2016) 'Mental health, mental illness and disability.' In Nicholson, A., McKimm, J. and Allen, A.K. (eds) *Global Health*. Sage.

Davies, J. (2013) *Cracked: why psychiatry is doing more harm than good.* Icon Books.

Dawson, S., Bierce, A., Feder, G. *et al.* (2021) Trauma-informed approaches to primary and community mental health care: protocol for a mixed-methods systematic review. *British Medical Journal*, 11.

Goffman, E. (1990[1963]) *Stigma: Notes on the management of spoiled identity.* Penguin.

Golightley, M. and Goemans, R. (2017) *Social Work and Mental health*, 6th edition. Sage.

Goodman, B. (2015) *Psychology and Sociology in Nursing*, 2nd edition. Learning Matters.

Harrington, A. (2019) *Mind Fixers: psychiatry's troubled search for the biology of mental illness.* W.W. Norton and Company.

Larkin, M. (2013) *Health and Wellbeing Across the Life Course.* Sage.

Lee, Y. and Jang, K. (2019) Mental health of grandparents raising grandchildren: understanding predictors of grandparents' depression. *Innovation in Aging*, **3**(1): 282.

Matthews, D. (2019) Capitalism and mental health. *Monthly Review*, **70**(8): 49–62.

Mehta, D. (2020) The genetic double whammy – autoimmune and mental health disorders. *Brain, Behavior, and Immunity*, **89**: 7–8.

Morrall, P. (2009) *Sociology and Health: an introduction*, 2nd edition. Routledge.

National Collaborating Centre for Mental Health (2021) *The Improving Access to Psychological Therapies Manual.* Available at www.england.nhs.uk/publication/the-improving-access-to-psychological-therapies-manual or bit.ly/3ZDi0Cx (accessed 5 December 2022).

NHS England (2019) NHS Long Term Plan. Available at: www.longtermplan.nhs.uk/wp-content/uploads/2019/01/nhs-long-term-plan-june-2019.pdf or bit.ly/3ZFcTSv (accessed 5 December 2022).

NMC (2018) *The Code: professional standards of practice and behaviour for nurses, midwives and nursing associates.* Nursing and Midwifery Council.

Petruccelli, K., Davis, J. and Berman, T. (2019) Adverse childhood experiences and associated health outcomes: a systematic review and meta-analysis. *Child Abuse and Neglect,* 97: 104127.

Pilgrim, D. and McKeown, M. (2018) 'Sociological understandings of mental health'. In Wright, K. and McKeown, M. (eds) *Essentials of Mental Health Nursing.* Sage.

Porter, E. (2013) *Madness: a brief history.* Oxford University Press.

Rogers, A. and Pilgrim, D. (2021) *A Sociology of Mental Health and Illness,* 6th edition. Open University Press.

Unicef (2020) *Worlds of Influence: understanding what shapes child well-being in rich countries.* Available at: www.unicef-irc.org/publications/1140-worlds-of-influence-understanding-what-shapes-child-well-being-in-rich-countries.html or bit.ly/3Zgu6Sd (accessed 22 December 2022).

Warner, R. (2004) *Recovery from Schizophrenia: psychiatry and political economy,* 3rd edition. Brunner-Routledge.

WHO (2004) *Promoting Mental Health: concepts, emerging evidence, practice.* World Health Organization. Available at: https://apps.who.int/iris/handle/10665/42940 (accessed 5 December 2022).

WHO (2022) *Depression.* World Health Organization. Available at: www.who.int/news-room/fact-sheets/detail/depression (accessed 5 December 2022).

9 LEARNING DISABILITY
Josh Hodgson

This chapter relates to outcomes 1.1, 1.2, 1.3, 1.4, 1.9, 1.10, 1.11, 2.1, 2.2, 2.4, 2.6, 2.7, 3.21, 3.22, 4.1 and 6.3 within the *Standards of Proficiency for Nursing Associates* (NMC, 2018).

LEARNING OUTCOMES

When you have completed this chapter you should be able to:
- Outline the theories of additional learning needs and challenging behaviours for both adults and children.
- Describe person-centred care.
- Discuss effective interventions that promote positive wellbeing for service users.
- Discuss the legislative and ethical frameworks within which provision is delivered and to which professionals must adhere.

9.1 Introduction

This chapter will introduce you to supporting people with a learning disability and explore some of the issues commonly encountered by people themselves and by those who support them, as well as issues surrounding contemporary learning disability practice. We will start by exploring the broad picture and needs of people with a learning disability and then break these down into more specific topics with the exploration of underpinning theory around these needs. We will also explore some practical solutions to overcome barriers you might encounter in practice when supporting someone with learning disabilities.

9.2 Learning disability – the broad picture

ACTIVITY 9.1A

Before reading on, consider what you already know about people with a learning disability. For example:
- Do you know of any models of disability; if so, which ones and what do they say?
- What is a learning disability and how is it diagnosed?
- What causes learning disability?

The label of 'learning disability' has been used since the late 1990s (Mitchell, 2019) and is currently the accepted term in most of the UK by people with a learning disability themselves. The care, support and image of people with a learning disability has changed significantly since the turn of the century. Once termed 'mental defectives' and banished to Victorian-style institutions, people with a learning disability were kept behind closed doors and 'relieved' of their burden on society (Mitchell, 2019).

Models and approaches to healthcare have evolved over the decades owing to developments in evidence-based practice, advances in capabilities and a more progressive change in attitudes towards people with a learning disability. Once upon a time the medical model was considered an appropriate model of care whereby the focus was on 'cure' and physical illness, to the general exclusion of most other things (including choice, inclusion and psychological needs). The emphasis the medical model placed was on the impairment or defect (what is wrong with the person) and blame placed there (Scope, 2020).

Fast forward in time to the emergence of the social model. The social model of disability, rather than placing blame onto the person for their impairments, emphasises that society places barriers which disable the person (disability, its meaning and definition is thereby socially constructed). *Table 9.1* puts these models in context.

Table 9.1 *Models of disability*

The medical model	The social model
The medical model might identify that someone with a learning disability has a cognitive defect and therefore the problem lies here. They cannot understand the world around them directly because of this cognitive problem and therefore this is the origin of their disability.	The social model, conversely, would identify that while a cognitive problem might exist, the world around the person needs to change and adapt to their needs and therefore the problem does not lie solely with the person but in the response of the world around them.

The biopsychosocial model (read more about this in *Chapter 5*) builds on how we consider health and wellbeing even more. The emphasis of the biopsychosocial model (indicated in the name) is on a multitude of factors and recognises that the person has biological, psychological and social needs. What this model does differently is that it recognises the effects each aspect of the person has on another and that needs coexist. For example, it recognises that there is a link between one's physical and mental health and wellbeing (in that one affects the other and therefore both sets of needs coexist and need to be addressed). In terms of this model, it recognises that a learning disability cannot be cured, and therefore we're looking at optimising the person's quality of life according to their wishes and considering their specific needs, rather than trying to find a cure or 'writing someone off', and doing so in a holistic, person-centred way (Wade and Halligan, 2017).

The first thing to remember about a person with a learning disability is that they are a person first, living with a diagnosis and this should not define them. Diagnostic labels can be useful tools to enable access to vital services, funding and support; however, they must be used with caution and person-centredness should always come first. Broadly speaking, learning disability is an umbrella term and a diagnostic label. In general, a person with a learning disability is likely to struggle with:

- Understanding and being understood by others
- Processing new and/or complex information
- Sudden change
- Keeping themselves safe
- Self-managing their health and social care needs.

In general, a person will be classed as having a learning disability if the following are satisfied:

- Full scale intelligence quotient (FSIQ) below 70 points, and;
- Problems in at least two areas of adaptive function (see below), and;
- This is diagnosed during childhood (up to 18 years of age), and;
- It has an enduring effect (lifelong).

The severity of a learning disability can vary across a spectrum and will differ from person to person. Simply knowing where a person's diagnosis is on the spectrum of mild to profound may help to anticipate needs to a degree, but this will be on an individual basis. IQ scores are shown in *Table 9.2*; bear in mind that it can be difficult to accurately assess profound learning disability.

Table 9.2 *Levels of learning disability severity*

Severity	IQ	General picture
Mild	50–69	Likely to have good levels of independence including potentially living alone and having a job May only require support with more complex situations (housing, bills, health needs) Requires complex information to be simplified
Moderate	35–49	Likely to require some level of support in daily life, in specific areas Likely to be able to communicate most needs
Severe	20–34	Likely to need support in most areas of daily living Likely to struggle with simple reading and writing
Profound and multiple	Below 20 or undetermined	Likely to be non-verbal Anticipation and meeting of all needs required Likely to require 24-hour care and support Unlikely to be able to meet any of own needs

Adapted from Vahabzadeh *et al.* (2011) and Barber (2022)

Adaptive function refers to one's ability to adapt to change or the challenges of daily life. For example:

You take the same bicycle route to work every day. One day, one of the roads is closed, meaning you need to take a diversion and go around your normal route. You manage this because you know the area well enough and simply take the next street around and return to your usual route thereafter.

A person with a learning disability may struggle to adapt to this change and to use judgement to problem-solve. This is an example of adaptive function.

The origin of a person's learning disability must be either pre- or post-natal. Generally speaking, this is diagnosed during childhood (for example, as a result of a parent noticing that a child has missed developmental milestones such as learning to walk, speak or toilet-train). Learning disability can sometimes be diagnosed in adulthood and this can be for reasons such as the person developing very good coping strategies, having a robust family support network around them or concealing their difficulties. A learning disability cannot be diagnosed after childhood if the origin relates to cognitive impairment as a result of an injury (such as a road traffic accident), as this will be classified as an acquired brain injury or cognitive impairment rather than a learning disability.

A learning disability can be caused by:
- Another condition or diagnosis (secondary to another condition)
- Parental lifestyle factors affecting the foetus (such as substance or alcohol misuse)
- Complications during pregnancy
- Complications at birth (such as hypoxia)
- Illness or injury during childhood
- Genetic and chromosomal abnormalities (such as trisomy 21, otherwise known as Down syndrome)
- Unknown causes (idiopathic).

A learning disability is diagnosed by a psychologist (often an educational psychologist or a clinical psychologist) who carries out a diagnostic assessment called a Wechsler Intelligence Scale for Children (if in childhood) or a Wechsler Adult Intelligence Scale (if in adulthood) which on completion provides a cognitive profile of the person to help determine their full-scale IQ and adaptive function.

Additional considerations in conjunction with a diagnosis of learning disability are:
- More/complex physical health problems
- Mental ill health
- Sensory impairments or difficulties
- Genetically predisposed conditions
- Comorbidities of a diagnosis.

The median age of death for someone with:
- A learning disability is 58
- Profound and multiple learning disability is 41
- Mild or moderate learning disability is 63.

The Learning Disability Mortality Review Programme (LeDeR) examined the deaths of people with a learning disability and found:
- Almost a third of deaths (31%) had underlying causes related to diseases of the respiratory system.
- Around 16% of deaths were related to diseases of the circulatory system.
- Sepsis, pneumonia and aspiration pneumonia are the leading causes of death in people with a learning disability (University of Bristol, 2019).
- People with a milder learning disability have a higher-than-average proportion of deaths associated with substance misuse due to differing lifestyle factors (Lakhan *et al.*, 2019).

Common myths:
1. A learning difficulty and a learning disability are the same thing – this is not correct. A difficulty is a specific learning need (such as dyslexia, dyscalculia or dyspraxia) with very specific needs. A learning disability is a global cognitive impairment.
2. Autism spectrum disorder (and conditions associated with the autistic spectrum) is a learning disability. While people with a learning disability are diagnosed with autism spectrum disorders at a higher prevalence than the general population and vice versa, they are not the same thing. Autistic people are supported by a range of services including learning disability services and also mental health services.

ACTIVITY 9.1B

Now revisit the questions at the beginning of this chapter in *Activity 9.1A* and match your knowledge against what you thought you knew and what you now know.

9.3 Comorbidities

ACTIVITY 9.2

As an illustration, we will shortly look at Down syndrome as a condition with a variety of comorbidities. Without looking this up and before moving on, consider what you already know about people with this condition. Do other conditions often accompany it? What might people with Down syndrome struggle with?

People with a learning disability, being part of the general population, experience the same health conditions as you or me, but they tend to have a much higher prevalence of these conditions, inequalities and issues. There are a number of reasons for this:

- People may struggle to identify when they feel unwell or alert others to this.
- Health and social care professionals may not possess the required level of education or understanding to support someone with a learning disability.
- Health or social care services may not be effectively adapted or adjusted to enable someone to access them.
- There is a higher rate of and genetic predisposition to other health conditions.
- There are commonly associated conditions owing to the nature of the effect learning disability has on the brain and body.

Conditions such as epilepsy, diabetes and mental health problems are significantly more common in people with a learning disability compared to other groups in the general population. A person with Down syndrome is a good example of the potential for complex needs and comorbidities.

Caveat: Always remember individual differences. Not everyone with a particular condition will be the same; this includes how learning disability affects someone and how every condition is experienced.

A person with Down syndrome is significantly more likely to develop issues around:

- Sight impairment
- Hearing impairment
- Enlarged tongue / reduced oral cavity
- Dysphagia (mechanical swallowing difficulty)
- Early onset dementia (around the age of 40 onwards)
- Coronary heart disease
- Congenital heart defects
- Hypothyroidism
- Coordination and motor impairments
- Respiratory conditions and diseases
- Epilepsy
- Obesity and weight management issues.

In taking a lifespan approach, also remember that conditions, symptoms and issues affect people differently and have an impact depending on where someone is on the lifespan.

For example, a congenital heart problem (congenital meaning a condition someone is born with, rather than developing later on) affects the way the heart works either because it has not developed properly, or a fault has developed with one of its functioning parts. In a child whose body has not fully developed, a condition like this might affect their growth and development, or they may develop other conditions because of the congenital defect which affect their health in other ways (such as problems with their blood pressure, other parts of their heart or other organs such as the lungs). The impact of a health condition on a growing and developing child is likely to be more significant simply because of the ability of their body to cope with problems compared to a fully developed adult.

Equally, conditions affecting older adults compared to working-age adults are likely to have a much more significant impact owing to the stage and state the body might be in during older age. Similarly to children, respiratory problems pose a more significant risk to young and older generations owing to the body's resilience and ability to cope with illness. In an older adult (who is already more likely to experience poorer health associated with age), the impact of a respiratory infection or issues such as Covid-19 are much more serious.

If we add into the mix that a younger, working-age or older person also has a learning disability (who we know are at much higher risk of poorer health) then the risk factors increase even further, requiring more care, attention and anticipation of need.

9.4 Capacity

Fact or myth?: everybody with a learning disability lacks capacity.

> **ACTIVITY 9.3**
>
> To help you answer the 'fact or myth' above and before reading on, consider:
> - What you already know about how a learning disability affects someone's understanding
> - What you already understand about the term 'capacity'
> - Whether you think learning disability might affect someone's capacity, and how.
>
> Bonus question: what other conditions or circumstances might affect capacity?

Capacity (or mental capacity) is simply the ability to make and communicate your own decisions. Many things might affect a person's capacity and the ability to make a decision around something in their life. In healthcare, we typically refer to making decisions around health, care or living arrangements (though there are many other decisions that can be considered). Lasting conditions affecting a person's cognition – such as a learning disability, acquired brain injury, cerebrovascular accident (CVA, or stroke) – or degenerative conditions such as dementia can all affect capacity and the ability to make a decision (this is illustrated a little more in the 'stage two assessment' below). Other more temporary conditions or states of mind can alter capacity, or at least make it fluctuate or vary. These might include intoxication (through illicit substances or alcohol), unconsciousness caused by an accident or early stages of conditions such as Alzheimer's disease.

There can be common misconceptions of capacity and consent in people with a learning disability. Examples of this include where blanket applications of capacity or incapacity have been imposed and have therefore led to poor, abusive and dangerous practices. This can include closed cultures like learning disability care where people may be less able to self-advocate or are less likely to be listened to and believed. It is important to remember that any service that delivers care can have a closed culture. It is never acceptable to assume incapacity, nor apply it across all of a person's decisions. The Mental Capacity Act (MCA) (2005) is the governing legislation which sets out the law in relation to someone who may lack capacity, and its Code of Practice identifies how to act within this piece of legislation and how to support someone.

The principles of capacity are:
1. Assume a person has capacity unless proven otherwise.
2. Do not treat people as incapable of making a decision unless all practicable steps have been tried to help them.
3. A person should not be treated as incapable of making a decision just because their decision may be unwise.
4. Always do things or take decisions for people without capacity in their best interests.
5. Before doing something to someone or making a decision on their behalf, consider whether the outcome could be achieved in a less restrictive way.

If someone is suspected to lack capacity concerning a specific decision, a two-stage assessment must be undertaken to determine whether they do actually lack capacity. This looks as follows:

Stage 1 assessment

Does the person have an impairment of their mind or brain, whether as a result of an illness, or external factor such as alcohol or drug use?

If the answer is yes, we can then move on to stage two below. If the answer to the above is no, we cannot therefore determine that the person lacks capacity around a decision.

Stage 2 assessment

Does the impairment mean the person is unable to make a specific decision when they need to?

The MCA identifies that people are unable to make a decision if they cannot:
1. Understand the information relevant to the decision (we might have to provide someone with information in an accessible format)

2. Retain the information (while also allowing someone time to process and respond to information)
3. Use or weigh up that information as part of the process of making the decision.

ACTIVITY 9.4

Before moving on, consider what you know about the following concepts in relation to capacity:

- Unwise decisions
- Restrictive practices
- Deprivations of liberty.

How would you determine if a decision fits into one of these categories?

Whether a person has capacity or not, it is always up to us to provide someone with information in a way they understand (which also relates to point number 1, above), to facilitate someone making an informed decision and to respect their needs and wishes in the least restrictive way possible (NHS, 2018). We also must be mindful that where a decision may be unwise, we understand what that means. Ultimately, an unwise decision is something we would not advocate, but the person has the capacity to make that decision. If a person *lacks capacity*, we should still take into account their opinions and perspectives even when acting in their best interests (SCIE, 2011).

9.4.1 Restrictive intervention

Where we need to consider something like a restrictive intervention (for example, where someone lacking capacity wants access to something, but we need to prevent it), again we must understand what that means and what the remit is. Restrictive interventions are deliberate acts on the part of other people that restrict a person's movement, liberty and/or freedom to act independently in order to:

- Take immediate control of a dangerous situation where there is a real possibility of harm to the person or others if no action is undertaken, and
- End or significantly reduce the danger to the person or others (HM Government, 2015).

Restrictive practice is making someone do something they do not want to do or stopping someone doing something they want to do (Skills for Health, 2011), otherwise known as a deprivation of liberty (SCIE, 2015; Idris and Mloyi, 2016). A justified deprivation of liberty, otherwise known as a deprivation of liberty safeguard, occurs when it is necessary to deprive the liberty of a resident or patient who lacks capacity to consent to their care and treatment in order to keep them safe from harm. The deprivation of liberty is seen as a last resort and involves the application to the 'supervisory body for authorisation' (the local authority in England, local health board for hospitals in Wales and local authority for care homes in Wales). The deprivation of liberty is not the same as someone being detained under the Mental Health Act (1983, 2007) whereby a person is prevented from leaving a ward or compelled to take treatment due to severe mental ill health. Being 'detained' or 'sectioned' is a compulsion to engage with medical assessment and/or treatment (SCIE, 2015).

>> **Deprivation of liberty is a last resort.**

A deprivation of liberty is likely to occur where there is a level of risk associated with something. A risk by definition is something which has the potential to cause harm or damage, and we may determine whether something is a risk by using some kind of assessment tool. Typically, these might have you explore an activity in relation to its potential for harm by looking at the severity of consequence if something goes wrong, multiplied by the likelihood of it going wrong. These often generate numerical risk categories which help you to determine how risky something is and therefore what level of mitigation or management you need to put into place as a result.

Risks can be reasonable, and these are usually whereby the benefit of the activity or decision outweighs the cost (risk). An example of this might be when supporting someone with road safety. There is an inherent risk with crossing the road, and to properly promote someone's autonomy to do something themselves (which is also called actively supporting someone – doing with, not for), there will be a point where there is still a risk of something going wrong, but the person needs to demonstrate crossing the road safely on their own (the benefit outweighs the risk). This is also called positive risk-taking, which is the practice of actively facilitating taking a calculated and reasonable risk for the benefit of the person's care, treatment and wellbeing, and according to their level of capacity (Skills for Care, 2011).

9.5 Communication

ACTIVITY 9.5

Reflect before moving on:

Consider the last time you supported somebody with a communication problem. What about it made it challenging for the person, and how did you adapt to this? What skills did you use?

Communication is one of the most important skills in health and social care practice. If we consider the medical versus social model of care mentioned earlier, we should take the stance that it is we as people and a society around the person who need to adapt our communication and make it accessible (the person's disability is not the problem).

A person with a learning disability might experience problems with communication, such as:

- Problems speaking (expressive: mechanically or dysphasia)
- Problems understanding speech (receptive: mechanically or dysphasia)
- Hearing problems
- Sight impairments
- Problems understanding or processing complex or more simplified language (spoken or written).

Health literacy is a specific issue in communication, affecting people with and without a learning disability, and is the ability to understand information related to one's own health, decisions around one's health, and making sense of information (such as written documents). Health literacy in people with a learning disability can differ for many reasons, including:

- Reading and writing abilities
- Level of schooling and formal qualifications (such as GCSEs or functional skills)
- Socioeconomic or demographic background
- Cognitive impairment
- Sensory impairments.

One of the most common frustrations people with a learning disability report is understanding what others say to them and expressing themselves verbally. It is up to us as professionals to adapt our communication systemically, rather than focus on people's deficits or impairments and as such, we can make simple 'reasonable adjustments' such as:

- Reduce staged commands (how many things we ask someone to do in a sentence, for example: 'please come in, sit yourself down and remove your coat' contains three commands in one sentence)
- Paraphrase (be concise, rephrase something more complex)
- Use simple terminology, words and phrases
- Reduce jargon
- Avoid being too abstract (English language, colloquialisms and 'reading between the lines' are all complexities that someone might struggle with. For example, avoid likening something to something else – say what you mean)
- Check understanding through repetition (repetition and rehearsal aid understanding)

- Modify the question to check understanding (ask the same question in more than one way to check if the person has understood, but do not use this as a method to 'catch someone out' as this is unethical)
- Speak slowly and clearly
- Be mindful of tone of voice (word choice accounts for about 8% of what people understand; tone of voice, body language and non-verbal cues account for about 92% of how people interpret and figure out what you are saying)
- Be mindful of your body language (reduce outward movements, be self-aware of eye contact and sitting position)
- Give time to process information and respond
- Provide easy-read documents
- Use the terminology or slang the person does (speaking in their language).

All of these are reasonable adjustments considered under the Equality Act 2010 (HM Government, 2010).

Adjusting the environment can also be considered and counts as a reasonable adjustment. People with a learning disability may have different sensory needs, preferences and dislikes to people you may otherwise support.

ACTIVITY 9.6

Consider the following scenario and identify what about the environment could be contributing factors:

You are working in a busy GP surgery running a small clinic. The clinic is brightly lit, very light-coloured and located in a busy corridor. You can hear some traffic from the road just outside and can often hear people in the waiting room when it's very busy. Your consulting room is relatively small with a desk, bed, computer and drawers of clinical equipment. There is a window at the furthest end, then your desk, two chairs for patients and the door.

Things you might have commented on which you could reasonably adjust might include:
- Lighting
- Doors and windows being open or closed
- Room layout
- Seating position in the room.

RECAP

- A person with a learning disability is a person first, living with a diagnosis.
- The severity of learning disability can vary across a spectrum.
- People with a learning disability are part of the general population and experience the same health conditions as people who do not have a learning disability, but they tend to have a much higher prevalence of these conditions, inequalities and issues.
- A person with a learning disability should be assumed to have capacity unless proven otherwise. If lack of capacity is suspected concerning a specific decision, a two-stage assessment must be undertaken to determine whether they do actually lack capacity.

9.6 The role of behaviour

ACTIVITY 9.7

Consider the following:

If you think about somebody whose behaviour might be described as 'challenging', what is it about that behaviour that is challenging? Who does it challenge and why?

If you are already working or on placement in a health or social care setting, think about the kinds of 'challenging' behaviour you might come across in your own practice, and for bonus points consider how you might prevent them from occurring in the first place or support the person if/when they do occur. Once you have read this chapter, return to this activity and compare notes on how you approached it before and after.

Behaviour is a form of communication in all of us; this is not exclusive to people with a learning disability. A behaviour has a function (why) and a topography (what). A behaviour may have more than one function but can be divided into social attention, tangible, escape or sensory (Cooper, Heron and Heward, 2007). The function of a behaviour refers to the source of environmental reinforcement for it (positive or negative) (Tarbox *et al.*, 2009). Without understanding the function of a behaviour, any intervention put in place could be ineffective and/or make the behaviour worse (O'Neill *et al.*, 1997).

Briefly, every behaviour (including your own!) has a function and serves to communicate some need or another:

- Sensory/stimulation (pain, too much stimulus)
- Social attention (laughing, gaining reaction from others)

- Tangible/activity (becoming excited, obtaining an item or gaining access to something)
- Escape/maintain (self-injury, resulting in avoiding doing something; or screaming to avoid ending a task/someone leaving).

These are basic functions of behaviour and should only be treated as such and should never be used to define or describe a person. Behaviour is much more complex and subtle in reality, including often having more than one function, and there is always a person involved and behind the behaviour. Undesirable behaviours can provide challenges to the person exhibiting them or to those around them.

Behaviour can be described as challenging when it is of such an intensity, frequency or duration as to threaten the quality of life and/or the physical safety of the individual or others and it is likely to lead to responses that are restrictive, aversive or result in exclusion (Royal College of Psychiatrists, British Psychological Society, Royal College of Speech and Language Therapists, 2007).

The definition of challenging behaviour can help us to identify when a behaviour might be considered challenging and involves comprehensive assessment to determine the function in order to support the person where required. The interesting aspect of this definition is the emphasis on the response of people toward the person exhibiting the behaviour.

A few terms you may come across in behavioural psychology are:
- Positive reinforcement – the introduction of a desirable stimulus after a behaviour which makes it more likely that behaviour will happen again
- Positive reward – a desirable stimulus provided to encourage the behaviour (for example, pocket money for doing housework)
- Positive punishment – an undesirable stimulus (punitive punishment) provided to discourage the behaviour (for example, telling someone off for doing something)
- Negative reinforcement – the removal of a stimulus designed to discourage the behaviour (for example, taking away access to a gaming console as a result of bad behaviour)
- Proactive strategies – steps put into place to avoid the behaviour occurring in the first place (for example, providing meaningful activity to prevent someone being bored or reducing stimulus in the environment as a matter of course to prevent someone becoming overwhelmed)
- Reactive strategies – steps put into place to intervene when a behaviour is happening or proactive strategies have not been effective (examples may include removing someone from the environment, use of medication or physical intervention).

In any intervention, irrespective of what it is, the following must be observed: use the least restrictive approach for the least amount of time using the least amount of force.

Any strategies should be carefully documented in a positive behaviour support plan and should be done in a person-centred, multidisciplinary way to ensure practices are

 Positive reward is the most effective way of reinforcing behaviour.

safe. As an absolute rule: positive reward is the most effective way of reinforcing behaviour. Positive punishment is wholly unacceptable and is not advocated in contemporary practice; use of positive punishment constitutes abusive practices and can result in safeguarding incidents. Negative reinforcement is somewhat effective, though the link between removal of stimulus as a reinforcer can be trickier for someone to understand compared to positive reward. Negative reinforcement is, however, often part of a positive behaviour support plan.

> **RECAP**
> - Behaviour is a form of communication and has a purpose
> - Positive reward is the most effective way to reinforce behaviour
> - Use the least restrictive approach in any intervention, for the least amount of time using the least amount of force.

9.7 Mental health

All of us have mental health, and people with a learning disability are no different. Around 25–40% of people with a learning disability experience mental health problems, which is higher than the figure associated with the population as a whole. Some will have a dual diagnosis (learning disability and mental health condition), and some will experience mental health as the population as a whole does (an episode in their lifetime). As with other conditions, a person with a learning disability may encounter additional difficulties if experiencing mental ill health. Reasons for this might include struggling to articulate if something is wrong or knowing how or when to seek help.

Individuals with a learning disability may also have a delay in developing emotional intelligence (desires, emotional regulation, self-awareness). As individuals without a learning disability, we are generally able to interpret emotions and understand what we are feeling and why. Someone with a learning disability may require some time and space to understand this. All too often individuals with a learning disability are forced and expected to manage with the change of environment around them and this has the potential to trigger an overwhelming array of emotions that the individual may struggle with. This causes the individual's protective instincts to activate, by physically expressing confusion, absent thinking and sometimes aggression (see functions of behaviour, above).

> **ACTIVITY 9.8**
>
> Take a moment to consider the mental health conditions or problems you know about already (see *Chapter 8*). Given what you know about them, do you think the symptoms of them might affect someone with a learning disability differently? How would you support someone with a learning disability to understand their mental health and wellbeing?

9.8 Contemporary initiatives and drivers for change

Many initiatives and drivers for change or specific attention exist within learning disability practice:

- Overmedication and polypharmacy (the prescription of four or more drugs in adults and two or more drugs in children) is a problem experienced by all, including people with a learning disability. The STOMP (Stopping the Over-Medication of People with a learning disability) campaign was launched in 2016. While most campaigns like this will focus generally on reducing the number of medicines people are prescribed – due to things like risk factors (such as increased falls risk, for example) or the increased likelihood of experiencing side-effects or interactions from other medicines – the STOMP initiative specifically focuses on the prescription of psychotropic drugs in people with a learning disability. Historically, people with a learning disability have been prescribed drugs such as antipsychotics (drugs used to alleviate symptoms of psychosis) and anxiolytics (drugs used to alleviate symptoms of anxiety or agitation) purely to 'manage' their behaviour and, more alarmingly, in the absence of a diagnosed mental health condition. Drugs like these may be used appropriately in a lot of circumstances; however, the standard is that there should be a clinically justifiable reason for their prescription (as with any drug).
- Since the CIPOLD Review (the Confidential Inquiry into the Premature deaths of People with a Learning Disability), questions have been raised in acute healthcare, particularly about the treatment of people with a learning disability accessing mainstream health services, and specifically around avoidable deaths. In response to avoidable and preventable deaths occurring in people with a learning disability, the LeDeR (Learning Disability Mortality Review) programme was devised with a primary function to review any reported death of someone with a learning disability and determine whether the cause or factors leading up to the death were preventable.

- The introduction of mandatory awareness training around people with a learning disability and/or autism will become available in early 2023 and was promoted by the widely publicised death of Oliver McGowan and the resulting campaigning by Paula McGowan (Oliver's mother). Oliver was wrongly administered an antipsychotic medication which he had reacted poorly to in the past (drug sensitivity) and as a result experienced a rare reaction called neuroleptic malignant syndrome. He developed encephalopathy and died as a result, diagnostic overshadowing being a major factor in his death. Diagnostic overshadowing occurs when health professionals assume that the behaviour of a person with learning disabilities is part of their disability, without exploring other potential causes such as biological factors. Nursing associates have a crucial role in reducing diagnostic overshadowing, ensuring that health professionals see the person and not just their disability.
- *Transforming Care* and the Winterbourne Enquiry (and subsequent Whorlton Hall Inquiry) are still widely discussed in learning disability practice. Institutional and abusive practices in assessment and treatment units sparked the inquiry and scrutiny into these services in 2011. While assessment and treatment units serve a specific purpose and should be used where required for short periods of assessment or treatment, care and treatment reviews (CTR) now exist to a) justify the need for someone to remain in hospital and b) to prevent admission to hospital where possible.

"People with learning disability start off as children, grow into adulthood and old age, get sick occasionally, have mental health problems more often than the rest of us, and some of them – whisper it – even need the services of the midwife." (McClimens and Burns, 2016, p. 29).

The reason that quote resonates so well is that it highlights that people with a learning disability essentially have the same needs as the rest of us and are people, part of the general population. What this chapter highlights is that while this is absolutely the case, we simply need to get better at making the reasonable adjustments to meet their needs more effectively, efficiently and with a bit of understanding.

9.9 Building a resource toolkit

The NMC standards indicate that you should not practise outside the scope of your competence and should seek support and make referrals where necessary. There are several ways you can start to develop your own resources and toolkits:

- Know who your learning disability champion or liaison is, how and when to contact them.
- Know which tools are useful in which circumstances and how to use them.

- Know where to look for further support, ideas, information and reasonable adjustments.

9.9.1 Liaison nurses

Learning disability liaison nurses exist in most Integrated Care Systems now and are key resources for people with a learning disability and acute staff. Liaison nurses' roles and responsibilities vary but can include:

- Consultation and advice when someone with a learning disability is coming into hospital for planned or unplanned care
- Direct work with the person and/or their families or carers
- Providing education and training to enhance staff ability to provide safe, effective and reasonably adjusted support.

9.9.2 Hospital passports

These collaborative, person-centred and individualised documents have been around for many years now and are not exclusive to people with a learning disability (you might see passports specific to other conditions, such as multiple sclerosis or dementia). Hospital passports are working documents with explicit information about a person such as their likes, dislikes, regular medications, dietary habits, recent health visits or appointments, vital information about their conditions and key advice about how to support the person. The idea of a hospital passport is to reduce barriers to supporting someone when they enter primary care (and even when they go between other regular care environments) and increase consistency and quality of care. You should be able to find a typical template by searching on the NHS website or via any online search engine.

9.9.3 Social media forums

The responsible and professional use of social media forums such as Facebook, Twitter, etc. should as far as reasonably possible be encouraged. If used properly, they are excellent resources for support and are an almost unlimited source of knowledge. Popular learning disability nursing forums exist on these platforms and resources are often shared nationally (maintaining confidentiality, of course). For example, you may require an easy-read version of a clinical procedure or medical treatment. While it is possible to learn the skills to create easy-read versions of documents yourself, the chances are someone else has done it, and is willing to share it on this sort of platform.

9.9.4 Toolkits

Various pre-designed, reputable and evidence-based toolkits exist which aim to provide you with a wealth of resources. There are many examples of pre-built toolkits which you can keep, ready to use to support someone with a learning disability accessing your service, including:

- Annual health checks: www.england.nhs.uk/learning-disabilities/improving-health/annual-health-checks or bit.ly/3YrczWl
- Friendships, sexual relationships and marriage: https://wales.mencap.org.uk/sites/default/files/2018-05/Friendships%20Sexual%20Relationships%20and%20Marriage%20%28March%202018%29v2.pdf or bit.ly/3IW1U0h
- Keele University: https://aldhc.keele.ac.uk/wttk

9.9.5 Websites and charities

Charities and third sector organisations specifically focus on enhancing the quality of care and support and are excellent examples of being a fountain of knowledge. Charity websites contain a wealth of resources freely available, ranging from fact sheets and assessment tools to aide-memoires and evidence-based resources.

- Mencap website: www.mencap.org.uk
- Bild (British Institute of Learning Disabilities) website: www.bild.org.uk
- National Learning Disability Nursing Forum: https://learningdisabilitynurse.co.uk
- *Building the Right Support for People with a Learning Disability*: https://assets.publishing.service.gov.uk/government/uploads/system/uploads/attachment_data/file/1092537/Building-the-Right-Support-for-People-with-a-Learning-Disability-and-Autistic-People-Action-Plan-accessible.pdf or bit.ly/3SPT9Jw
- The LeDeR report into the avoidable deaths of people with learning disabilities: www.kcl.ac.uk/research/leder

9.9.6 Journals

Academic and peer-reviewed journals are a solid example of evidence-based resources and practice. Journals offer quality sources of evidence around issues facing people with a learning disability, evaluation of interventions, provision of people's stories and more.

9.10 The impact of Covid-19 on people with a learning disability

People with a learning disability often experience health inequalities more significantly than others in the general populus, and the pandemic highlighted that. During the pandemic, some of the major issues disproportionately affecting people with a learning disability have been:

Vaccinations: People with a learning disability were not initially counted as 'clinically extremely vulnerable' and therefore did not have immediate access to the vaccination programme. As we explored earlier, people with a learning disability have a higher incidence of health and wellbeing problems (such as respiratory and circulatory health problems) and thus increased vulnerability to viruses like SARS-Cov-2 (the coronavirus). This was altered eventually, and vaccinations were made more readily available.

Do Not Attempt Cardiopulmonary Resuscitation (DNACPR): Towards the beginning of the pandemic, DNACPRs were being issued to patients in hospitals much more readily and people with a learning disability were disproportionately being issued them, seemingly without clinical justification. A learning disability does not inherently determine the need to have a DNACPR in place; what should dictate that is clinical need and a balanced decision including the person and those around them. A decision would consider whether quality of life would diminish if CPR was successful, in the event of cardiopulmonary arrest. This practice was challenged nationally and changed, thankfully.

Mortality: Statistics published in November 2020 by Public Health England suggested that people with a learning disability were six times more likely to die with Covid-19 than the general population.

IMPORTANT NOTE! Aside from the specific impacts and challenges the pandemic presented to people with a learning disability, the after-effects described by much of the population still apply here. For example, mental health and wellbeing is more widely being talked about now and negative impacts were also felt by people with a learning disability (look back at *Section 9.7* on mental health). Additionally, considering what we know about the most common causes of death in people with a learning disability (diseases and disorders of the respiratory system), Covid-19 (and long Covid) may disproportionately affect the respiratory health of people with a learning disability.

ACTIVITY 9.9

Do some of your own research on the effects of acute Covid-19 infection and long Covid and consider the additional impacts this might have on a person with a learning disability.

9.11 Conclusion

We have explored a great range of topics and challenges faced by people with a learning disability and those who support them, looking at some pragmatic and simple solutions which can be implemented in practice to enhance the care and support of people with a learning disability. It is of course important to acknowledge that these are not exhaustive lists of needs and as we have reinforced in this chapter, people with a learning disability experience the same health and social care needs as the rest of the population. It is simply in the way in which we meet those needs that the difference lies, and the responsibility of adjusting practice to do that sits with us as healthcare professionals.

Aside from the transferable concepts – such as person-centredness, compassion and holism – practices which should remain at the forefront of all contemporary healthcare, particularly

>> **Remember above all that people with a learning disability are people first.**

while supporting people with a learning disability, include remembering that behaviour is a form of communication, least restrictive practices should always be followed, and we must be careful to avoid diagnostic overshadowing. Practising in this manner helps in reducing the health inequality gap disproportionately experienced by people with a learning disability and if followed properly, helps to maintain trust and safe practice.

CHAPTER SUMMARY

- A person with a learning disability is a person and should not be defined by their diagnosis.
- A person with a learning disability may have difficulties adapting to change and problem-solving.
- A person with a learning disability may experience the same health conditions as those found within the general population but with a higher prevalence.
- Nursing associates as health professionals need to adapt their communication to make it accessible to a person with a learning disability.
- Behaviour is a form of communication and positive reward is the most effective way to reinforce behaviour.
- A person with a learning disability is more likely to experience a mental health problem than members of the general population.

FURTHER READING

Barber, C. (2022) *Learning Disabilities: a non-specialist introduction for nursing, health and social care.* Lantern Publishing.

Health Education England (2019) *Core Capabilities Framework for Supporting Autistic People.* Available at: https://skillsforhealth.org.uk/wp-content/uploads/2020/11/Autism-Capabilities-Framework-Oct-2019.pdf or bit.ly/3F2d7LA (accessed 13 December 2022).

Langdon, P (2020) *COVID-19 and People with Learning Disabilities – challenging behaviour and mental health.* Available at: www.rcpsych.ac.uk/docs/default-source/events/presentations/webinars/langdon-peter.pdf?sfvrsn=5283f593_2 or bit.ly/3IVLDbB (accessed 13 December 2022).

Mitchell, D. (2019) A century of learning disability nursing. *Learning Disability Practice*, **22**(1): 11–13.

NHS (2017) *Next Steps on the NHS Five Year Forward View*. Available at: www.england.nhs.uk/wp-content/uploads/2017/03/NEXT-STEPS-ON-THE-NHS-FIVE-YEAR-FORWARD-VIEW.pdf or bit.ly/3L00vYZ (accessed 13 December 2022).

NHS (2019) *Long Term Plan: learning disability and autism*. Available at: www.longtermplan.nhs.uk/areas- of-work/learning-disability-autism or bit.ly/3ZmSrWt (accessed 13 December 2022).

Scope (2020) Social model of disability. Available at: www.scope.org.uk/about-us/social-model-of-disability/#:~:text=The%20medical%20model%20of%20disability,and%20control%20in%20their%20lives or bit.ly/3F3wuUn (accessed 13 December 2022).

Skills for Health, Health Education England and NHS England (2019) *Core Capabilities Framework for Supporting People with a Learning Disability*. Available at: www.skillsforhealth.org.uk/wp-content/uploads/2020/11/Learning-Disability-Framework-Oct-2019.pdf or bit.ly/3ISSu5F (accessed 13 December 2022).

University of Bristol (2019) *Learning Disability Mortality Review (LeDeR)*. Available at: www.bristol.ac.uk/media-library/sites/sps/leder/LeDeR_2019_annual_report_FINAL2.pdf or bit.ly/3ZqnC3j (accessed 13 December 2022).

References

Barber, C. (2022) *Learning Disabilities: a non-specialist introduction for nursing, health and social care*. Lantern Publishing.

Cooper, J., Heron, T. and Heward, W. (2007) *Applied Behaviour Analysis*. Pearson Education.

HM Government (2010) Equality Act.

Idris, A. and Mloyi, R. (2016) *Reducing Restrictive Practice*. Available at: www.england.nhs.uk/6cs/wp-content/uploads/sites/25/2016/07/reduc-restrictiv-practice.pdf or bit.ly/3IU9o3z (accessed 13 December 2022).

Lakhan, R., Sagiraju, H., Ekúndayò, O. and Sharma, M. (2019) Substance use disorder in people with intellectual disabilities: current challenges in low- and middle-income countries. *Journal of Neurosciences in Rural Practice*, **10**(2): 301–305.

McClimens, A. and Burns, S. (2016) Looking after service users part two: nursing versus social work. *Learning Disability Practice*, **19**(2): 27–30.

Mental Capacity Act (2005). HMSO.

NHS (2018) *Mental Capacity Act*. Available at: www.nhs.uk/conditions/social-care-and-support-guide/making-decisions-for-someone-else/mental-capacity-act or bit.ly/3mtZDli (accessed 13 December 2022).

NMC (2018) *Standards of Proficiency for Nursing Associates*. Nursing and Midwifery Council.

O'Neill, R., Horner, R., Albin, R. *et al.* (1997) *Functional Assessment and Programme Development for Problem Behaviour: a practical handbook*. Brooks/Cole Publishing Company.

Royal College of Psychiatrists, British Psychological Society and Royal College of Speech and Language Therapists (2007) *Challenging Behaviour – a unified approach*. Available at: www.rcpsych.ac.uk/docs/default-source/improving-care/better-mh-policy/college-reports/college-report-cr144.pdf?sfvrsn=73e437e8_2 or bit.ly/3kRlnai (accessed 13 December 2022).

SCIE (2011) *Mental Capacity Act: respecting the right to make unwise decisions*. Social Care Institute for Excellence. Available at: www.scie.org.uk/mca/practice/decision-making/unwise-decisions or bit.ly/3YmHGT2 (accessed 13 December 2022).

SCIE (2015) *Deprivation of Liberty Safeguards (DoLS) at a glance*. Social Care Institute

for Excellence. Available at: www.scie.
org.uk/mca/dols/at-a-glance (accessed 13
December 2022).

Skills for Care (2011) *Learning to Live with Risk.*

Tarbox, J., Wilke, A., Najdowski, A. *et al.*
*(*2009) Comparing indirect, descriptive,
and experimental functional assessments
of challenging behavior in children with
autism. *Journal of Developmental and
Physical Disabilities,* **21**: 493–514.

University of Bristol (2019) *Learning Disability
Mortality Review (LeDeR).* Available at:

www.bristol.ac.uk/media-library/sites/
sps/leder/LeDeR_2019_annual_report_
FINAL2.pdf or bit.ly/3ZqnC3j (accessed 13
December 2022).

Vahabzadeh, A.B.N., Delaffon, V., Abbas, M.
and Biswas, A.B. (2011) Severe learning
disability. *InnovAIT,* **4(2)**: 91–7.

Wade, D. and Halligan, P. (2017) The
biopsychosocial model of illness: a model
whose time has come. *Journal of Clinical
Rehabilitation,* **31**(8): 995–1004.

INDEX